REMARKABLE

WOMEN

—— *of the* ——

FINGER
LAKES

REMARKABLE

WOMEN

of the

FINGER
LAKES

Julie Cummins

THE
History
PRESS

Published by The History Press
Charleston, SC
www.historypress.com

Copyright © 2023 by Julie Cummins
All rights reserved

First published 2023

Manufactured in the United States

ISBN9781467150477

Library of Congress Control Number: 2022951591

CONTENTS

CONTENTS

PART III. INFLUENCERS

ACKNOWLEDGEMENTS

In appreciation to Blair, Banks Smither, Dr. Peter, Louise and Stephanie, who helped make it happen.

Many thanks,

Julie Cummins

INTRODUCTION

D oing research is like playing detective. First you dig for the easy-to-find surface facts, and then you dig deeper, hoping for those nuggets of anecdotes that add dimension to the individual.

Such was the case with Blanche Stuart Scott, the first woman to fly in America. I first discovered her on a visit to the Glenn Curtiss Museum in Hammondsport, New York. A large metal plaque cited all of the Early Bird pilots, those who flew before 1916, Blanche was just one of a handful of women listed. Hardly anyone seemed to have heard of her. The gift shop had only a commemorative stamp and a short, half-page bio. A light bulb moment turned on, and I wondered if there were other forgotten or overshadowed women who were somehow connected to the Finger Lakes. The search was on.

In research, one clue can lead to another. Sometimes you find a gem, while others end at a brick wall, or sometimes it pops up right in front of you. Clues can be misleading and sometimes conflicting.

Consider Pearl White. The internet kept showing her name as a car color. Also, when I checked out her most famous film, *The Perils of Pauline*, I found that the cinematographer was Arthur Miller. I jumped to the conclusion that it was *the* Arthur Miller who married Marilyn Monroe. After I searched further, it was obvious that the two men were not the same person. Different ages and the middle initial C. separated the two men.

Other times, paths cross unknowingly. For example, Mabel Patter Daggett (listed with the other names of too little information) and Maud Humphrey both worked at *The Delineator* magazine but at different times. One wonders if they knew each other.

So, how did I decide to include the twenty-one women who are in this book? My criteria were that each one had some link to one of the eleven Finger Lakes and was not well known—in some cases, barely known. All of them were born and lived in the 1800s and made a worthy contribution to women's history. They were strong women who overcame gender bias and should have recognition.

That framework then ruled out Susan B. Anthony, Clara Barton, Amelia Earhart and Mary Jameson, whose names were more well known. There were five women I wanted to include but couldn't find enough information about them to be included:

Harriet Adams (1843–?): Doctor, Palmyra
Lavinia Chase (1840–?): Interpreter for Congress, Palmyra
Mabel Patter Daggett (1871–1927): Author and editor, Syracuse
Emily Howland (1827–1929): Educator, Sherwood
Mary Jane Holmes (1825–1919): Novelist, Brockport

The eleven Finger Lakes all have Native American names. According to legend, they came into being when the Great Spirit placed the imprint of his hand in blessing on the Upstate land. Bodies of water, large and small, fascinate people, as evidenced by the popularity of the Finger Lakes. The list of lakes goes in the order of east to west:

Otisco
Skaneateles
Owasco
Cayuga
Seneca
Keuka
Canandaigua
Honeoye
Canadice
Hemlock
Conesus

Canadice has the smallest surface area at 649 acres, Seneca the largest at 21.8 square miles; Cayuga is the longest at 40 miles. Depths range from

30 feet in Honeoye to 276 in Canandaigua. The larger lakes are bound to generate legends of water serpents. Stories of sightings of one in Seneca Lake have survived for hundreds of years, like the Loch Ness monster. So far, no proof.

The lakes were a necessary method of travel for many of these women and a place of relaxation for others. So much of history is discovery, and I am delighted to bring to light these women and their accomplishments.

PART 1

WELLNESS

ELIZABETH BLACKWELL
(1821–1910), "MED EX"

Geneva

Elizabeth Blackwell had two strikes against her: she was a woman in the 1800s, and she wanted to work in the male-dominated field of medicine. But she was determined not to let either challenge stand in her way.

Elizabeth was born in Bristol, England, and had a happy childhood. Her loving parents held liberal attitudes about child-rearing and religion. If the children misbehaved, instead of beating them, their mother recorded their inappropriate behavior in her black book. Too many black marks, and the children might be exiled to the attic during dinner.

Elizabeth's father, Samuel, was equally liberal in his belief that each child, even the girls, should have a religious and academic education that fostered the development of each one's talents and skills. Elizabeth was the third of nine children and had not only a governess but also a private tutor for intellectual growth. As a result, she was more isolated from the rest of the family.

However, all of their liberal education and religious views didn't pay the bills, and the family found themselves in serious debt, prompting them to emigrate from England to New York City in 1832. Supposedly, it was due to the failure of the father's sugar refining business, but the real reason and underlying purpose of the move was so Samuel could pursue abolition activities. The family moved six years later to Cincinnati, Ohio, but hard times continued. When Elizabeth's father died at the age of forty-eight, he left the family in poverty. Each family member had to work to pay the debts.

Elizabeth and two of her sisters opened a private school that lasted for two years, but at age twenty-four, she decided she wanted to go into medicine. Yet she lacked the finances to do so. She took a position as a music teacher in an exclusive girl's school in South Carolina. She saved money for one year and accepted another teaching position in South Carolina so she would have access to a doctors' library to study medicine. She sent applications to twenty-nine medical schools and received twenty-eight rejections. One was sent to Dr. Joseph Warrington in Philadelphia, Pennsylvania, who discouraged her because he believed men should be doctors and women should be nurses—a common belief held by many.

This was just one of many challenges that Elizabeth would face in her lifetime. Her determination and persistence paid off when number twenty-nine offered acceptance to Geneva Medical School (forerunner of Hobart and William Smith College) in Geneva, New York. She studied hard in medical school in 1847 and was a disciplined student who was friendly toward her fellow classmates, in spite of harassment from resident male doctors who deliberately changed or hid her patients' charts. When the results of the final exams were announced, Elizabeth had the best academic record in her class. Her thesis on typhus was a major accomplishment. It was so well done that even the senior staff praised it, changing any minds who doubted her. Elizabeth had successfully achieved her goal.

On January 23, 1849, Elizabeth made history by becoming the first female doctor in the United States. At her graduation, she was the last one in line, setting her apart from the others. When the dean conferred her diploma, he stood up and bowed to her. She responded, "Sir, I thank you. It shall be the effort of my life to shed honor on your diploma," blushed and bowed to him, and the audience burst into applause. When Elizabeth left the ceremony, the local women who had previously snubbed her smiled and nodded.

Elizabeth was realistic about her fame, but she recognized the need for more training and went to Paris to work at a maternity hospital. The same female bias followed her. Then an accident happened. She was enrolled in a midwives' course at La Maternité. While she was there, she contracted an infectious eye disease that left her blind in one eye. Unfortunately, it forced her to give up hope of becoming a surgeon. It was yet another obstacle for her to overcome.

She returned to New York in the summer of 1851 in the hopes of finding a medical position; instead, she was refused posts in the city's hospitals and dispensaries. She was even unable to rent private consulting space, which meant her private practice was slow to develop.

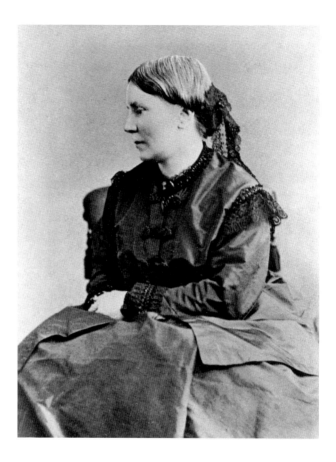

Portrait of Blackwell.
*Courtesy of Wikimedia
Commons.*

Meanwhile, she wrote a series of letters that were published in 1852 titled *The Laws of Life with Special Reference to the Physical Education of Girls*. A year later, those letters led to Elizabeth opening a small dispensary in a slum district. Her sister Dr. Emily Blackwell followed in her footsteps and joined her along with Dr. Marie Zakrzewska, another pioneer female doctor in the United States. In May 1857, the greatly enlarged dispensary was incorporated into the New York Infirmary for Women and Children.

Elizabeth never married but was fond of children. She adopted an Irish orphan, Kitty Barry, along with two dogs as her companions.

In 1859, during a yearlong lecture tour in Great Britain, recognition of Elizabeth's work began to spread. She became the first woman to have her name placed on the British medical register. Shortly after that, the American Civil War erupted, and Elizabeth helped organize a unit of field doctors called the Women's Central Association of Relief and trained nurses for war service.

At this point and time, another woman entered Elizabeth's life: the famous nurse Florence Nightingale. The two of them perfected a plan to create a medical school, and in 1868, the Women's Medical College in New York City was born. Elizabeth herself set the standards for admission, clinical training and certification as well as holding the chair of hygiene. The school operated for thirty-one years, becoming the New York–Presbyterian Lower Downtown Hospital in Manhattan.

In 1869, she moved permanently to England, where she established a successful private practice, helped organize the National Health Society and was appointed professor of gynecology at the London School of Medicine for Women. In 1907, another misfortune followed her. On vacation in Scotland, a crippling fall down a flight of stairs forced her to retire, but she continued to write and lecture until her death at the age of ninety-one.

Elizabeth was a pioneer who left behind a legacy of medical breakthroughs for women's rights. Among the many tributes to her is an annual award given by the American Medical Women's Association to a female physician. Most prominent is a full-size sculpture of her seated and holding a book in the midst of the city of Geneva where it all began. She was one of many women who dared to break gender barriers for the benefit of those who followed her.

CORDELIA GREENE
(1831–1905), "BOTTLED WATER"

Lyons

Could a woman be a doctor in the late 1800s? It was highly unlikely, as the primary and foremost occupation that was acceptable in those days was teaching. Yet Cordelia Greene would prove that wrong.

Her path to making medical history was rocky, confronting bias toward women, especially against female doctors, but her determination and passion prevailed.

Just before Cordelia was born, the family moved from New England to a site along the Erie Canal. Because Cordelia's parents had married outside the Quaker faith, Jabez Greene changed the family's religion from Quaker to Presbyterian.

She was one of five children and was greatly influenced by her parents, especially her father, Jabez. He was a farmer whose religious fervor was matched by his interest in progressive education. He carried out his convictions by serving as a trustee in the local public school and introducing the graded system. His beliefs and actions had a significant effect on Cordelia.

At age sixteen, she earned a teacher's certificate and taught in country schools long enough to earn money to put herself through medical school. The young teenage girl could have been a student herself, as some of her pupils were even taller than her. For her service, she received room and board and a salary of $3, which would be the equivalent of about $508 today, not much to live on. Nevertheless, it was sufficient to gain her enrollment in the Cleveland Medical School (later renamed Case Western

Reserve), where she was an excellent student. In 1853, she was the first woman to graduate with honors.

By happenstance, she read an article written by the renowned Elizabeth Blackwell, the first woman to become a doctor in the country. It became the turning point in Cordelia's life and the inspiration that she needed to pursue medicine as a career.

For practice, she worked long hours in the sanitarium that her father had purchased and opened as a small water cure facility in Castile, New York. She worked alongside him until he died and then took over his enterprise, using the natural sulfur springs as restorative treatment.

The hydrotherapy involved wrapping a cold, wet sheet pack around the patient with her arms straight at her sides. Then layers of woolen blankets were wrapped over the wet sheet pack from head to toe, completely swaddling the patient. The belief was that as the patient sweated, the secretions from her pores would be trapped in the sheet and the wool blankets would prevent moisture from evaporating into the air.

The water cure was the biggest draw for patients, but Cordelia believed in the importance of deep breathing, vigorous exercise and proper hydration of the body. She began every day by visiting patients' rooms and personally delivering a pitcher of water and ensuring that each one drank a full glass of water before breakfast.

Many of the patients who came to her had tried other doctors in hopes of curing their incapacitating headaches (now called migraines). When they first met Dr. Greene, they were surprised first that the doctor was a woman and second by her youthfulness. But they were quickly impressed with her healing methods.

The fame of the sanitarium spread across the country, and famous women flocked to her doors, including Susan B. Anthony, foremost suffragist; Frances Willard, founder of the Woman's Christian Temperance Union; and Dr. Clara Swain, credited with opening the first hospital for women in Asia.

Cordelia's life was far from typical. She never married and had no children of her own, but her nurturing nature led her to adopt six children. Despite those who may have raised their eyebrows, it was just one of the ways in which she dedicated her life to helping others. All of the children were given piano lessons, and the girls were instructed in household chores and the boys in carpentry. Each of the children was expected to maintain a garden and was given an apple tree of his or her own to cultivate. Family discussions at dinnertime were lively.

most dangerous time!   your nerves strong.

Dr. Greene's Nervura Blood and Nerve Remedy,

Guaranteed Purely Vegetable and Harmless, IS THE GREATEST AND BEST

Spring Medicine!

Are You Prepared for Spring?

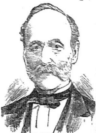

It is necessary to prepare yourself for the advent of spring by taking a spring medicine. Use the remedy which cured S. W. Nourse, Esq., of Hudson, Mass.

"From constant worry over business matters," he said, "I suffered from the loss of sleep, and became so nervous that I was entirely unfitted for my business. In fact, I feared insanity. I used Dr. Greene's Nervura blood and nerve remedy. The effect was almost magical. I could again sleep, mental composure, appetite, and strength returned. Six bottles of this remedy cured me, and I have remained well to this date. I have recommended Dr. Greene's Nervura blood and nerve remedy to many of my friends and neighbors, and have yet to learn of a failure to obtain good results."

He was Cured by Dr. Greene's Nervura Blood and Nerve Remedy.

S. W. NOURSE, Esq.

How to Get Well and Keep Well.

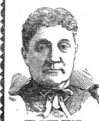

Do You Feel Weak, Tired, and Nervous?

The wonderful cure of Mrs. Oliver Wilson, of Northboro, Mass., will interest you.

"I was suffering from nervousness," she says, "caused by female weakness and nervous prostration. I was so nervous and weak I could not go up a common pair of stairs without stopping to rest, and was troubled to sleep at night. I took Dr. Greene's Nervura blood and nerve remedy, and have obtained my old elastic step around the home, to the surprise of my friends. After creeping around for two years, hardly able to do anything, it has proved a boon to me truly. I know of many others whom it has cured and who speak most highly in praise of it."

MRS. OLIVER WILSON.

Everybody Should take a Spring Medicine.

Read this and You Will Know What to Use.

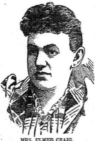

Mrs. Elmer Craig, of LeRoy, Ill., tells you how you can be well and strong:

"I was stricken with nervous disease," she says, "which affected my heart, head, and stomach. I doctored with physicians of our town, but got no relief from the terrible sick headaches, pains in the heart and stomach until I used Dr. Greene's Nervura blood and nerve remedy. Before I used this wonderful medicine the nerves in my eyes were so affected that I feared that I would lose my sight. I would run so nervous and weak I could not walk across the room without terrible palpitation of the heart. I had not taken one bottle of Dr. Greene's Nervura blood and nerve remedy before my head and eyes were cleared of their dull aching, and I am growing stronger every day. I cannot do half justice in the praise of this medicine."

MRS. ELMER CRAIG.

Is Your Blood Pure, Are Your Nerves Strong?

Mr. Seth E. Parsons, of 22 Park St., Albany, N. Y., one of Albany's most prominent business men, states:

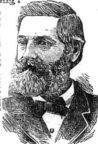

"I was very nervous. I could not hold my hands still, especially my left hand; there was an involuntary motion of the muscles and movement of the fingers. My food troubled me very much after eating. My kidneys and bladder were affected so it was difficult to urinate freely.

"I used the celebrated medicine, Dr. Greene's Nervura blood and nerve remedy, and without being tedious reciting my experience, I can say that these difficulties have left me, and my nerves are quiet and my food does not distress me. I feel without hesitation in saying that I think Dr. Greene's Nervura blood and nerve remedy has produced these favorable results."

Dr. Greene's Nervura Blood and Nerve Remedy Cured Him.

MR. SETH E. PARSONS.

To get well and to keep well, take

Dr. Greene's Nervura Blood and Nerve Remedy.

It is the discovery and Prescription of a successful Physician.

DR. GREENE, 35 West 14th St., New York City, can be consulted free, personally or by letter.

Advertisement for Dr. Greene's "spring medicine." *Author's collection.*

Her reputation quickly spread far and wide as a physician, suffragist and philanthropist. She played a significant role in all three causes. For many years, she refused to pay her taxes in order to protest her lack of the right to vote.

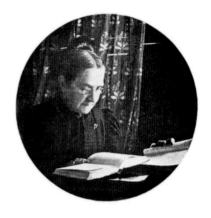

When her many fans and supporters asked her how she would like to celebrate her fiftieth birthday, her answer was: build a library. She donated the land in 1897 and provided $12,000 for an endowment. Plus, her many friends each gave $50, adding to the $500 of original stimulus money for books. Thus, the Castile Public Library was born—it still exists today.

Greene in a 1925 publication. *Courtesy of Wikimedia Commons.*

In 1904, Cordelia traveled to Washington, D.C., as the leading speaker of the National Woman's Christian Temperance Union convention. From there she went to New York City, where she became ill and never rallied.

Cordelia died in 1905, ironically from complications of emergency surgery. She strongly believed that one's years should be devoted to the encouragement and inspiration of others. Her medical achievements and support of women's rights did exactly that, paving the way for other women to follow.

ANNA CAROLINE MAXWELL (1851–1929), "AMERICAN NIGHTINGALE"

Bristol

Anna Caroline Maxwell seemed destined to be a nurse. Throughout her entire life, she was committed to training, mentoring and advancing the profession of nursing. She was a true pioneer who became known as the "American Florence Nightingale."

Little is known about her childhood other than she moved from the small town of Bristol, New York, to Canada with her family. When they moved back to the States in 1878, Anna settled in Boston and entered the Boston City Hospital, which was known as a training school for nurses. In 1880, she received her diploma, and that same year she was hired by Montreal General Hospital to implement a nursing program.

From there on, it was a fast track to a distinguished career.

In just a year's time, she was offered the position of superintendent of Massachusetts General Hospital's Training School for Nurses. What followed was a series of jobs, bouncing from one to another, but always with nurse training at the forefront of importance.

In 1889, she became the director of nursing at St. Luke's Hospital in New York City. Word spread about this accomplished nurse, and she was soon recruited by Presbyterian Hospital to oversee its new nursing school. The board president was determined to make Presbyterian the best hospital in not only New York City but the country as well. His first goal was hiring Anna as director. For her, the move there would be the most significant and lasting one of her life. She remained there until 1921.

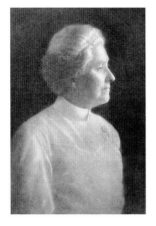

Portrait of Anna Maxwell.
Courtesy of Wikimedia Commons.

In 1892, Presbyterian became Columbia University School of Training. Student nurses worked and studied twelve hours a day, six days a week, for nine dollars a month. Two years later, twenty-one women were the first graduates.

Their experience and training would come into play in 1898, when Anna traveled to Georgia to treat soldiers in the Spanish-American War. She was faced with a grim scene of men suffering with typhoid, measles, yellow fever and malaria. She oversaw the nursing staff at the camp hospital, where one thousand patients were admitted but only sixty-seven died. It was there that she earned the title the "American Florence Nightingale," a tribute to the English nurse who treated wounded soldiers during the Crimean War

Anna became involved in a different kind of war, World War I. She lobbied on behalf of the nurses who had worked at the camp by making them commissioned officers, but it was an uphill battle. Due to the determination and perseverance of Anna and other nurse supporters they succeeded in petitioning Congress to create a nursing corps to care for soldiers at war. In 1901, the Army Nurse Corps was established along with officer ranking for military nurses.

She retired in 1921 and spent her time raising money for Columbia University's Anna C. Maxwell Hall, a residence for student nurses.

When she died in 1929, it was fitting that she was given full military honors in Arlington National Cemetery, the first woman to receive such recognition.

Among her many awards and accolades were founder of the *American Journal of Nursing*, active in recruiting nurses for military work through the Red Cross Nursing Service, coauthored with Amy Pope the book *Practical Nursing: A Textbook for Nurses* and active in the International Congress of Nursing. France awarded her the worldwide Public Health Medal and held a parade in her honor.

The footprints that Anna left behind were a legacy of setting standards for nursing education and recognition of nursing as a profession. Over a century after her death, the effects of her pursuit of excellence in nursing continue to be felt today. Thanks to Anna, many lives were saved. She revolutionized nursing and led the way.

MARY EDWARDS WALKER
(1832–1919), "SUIT YOURSELF"

Oswego

Mary Walker's name was not uncommon, but without a doubt her life and career were. She was the epitome of the independent woman of the Civil War era. Whether doctor, spy, prisoner of war, advocate for women's rights or defier of society rules, Mary was her own person.

Mary's parents, Alvah and Vesta Walker, believed their seven children, especially the six girls, should be educated. They were abolitionists and free thinkers who practiced nontraditional parenting roles. Her mother helped with the heavy labor on the family farm, and her father took over household chores. Mary didn't wear women's clothes, following her mother's belief that corsets and tight lacings were unhealthy. It was a cause that she practiced and pursued her entire life, wearing trousers, vest, coat and top hat. More than once, she was put in jail for impersonating a man.

To ensure that their children would be properly educated, Mary's parents started a local school. It was the first free schoolhouse in Oswego in the 1930s. After a primary education, Mary pursued medical sciences, and in 1855, she graduated as a medical doctor from Syracuse Medical College. She was the only woman in her graduating class.

That same year, she married fellow medical student Albert Miller. When it was time to say their vows, Mary typically refused to take his name or say the word *obey*. Instead of a gown, she wore a short skirt with trousers underneath, Bloomer style.

Mary and Albert went into private practice for a few years, but people were too leery of a female doctor and the Civil War had just started. What

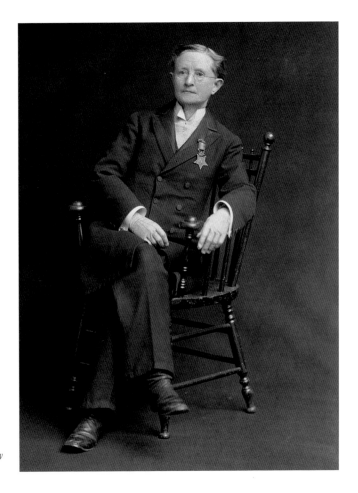

Dr. Mary Walker
with her Medal of
Honor, circa 1916.
*Courtesy of the Library
of Congress.*

Mary really wanted to do was to join the army as a surgeon. Even with her excellent credentials the military refused to bend the rules. No women were allowed to be doctors. But Mary had a way of getting around things; she volunteered for the Union army and was the only female doctor to provide medical service to Union soldiers. Despite that, she was refused a commission as an army surgeon. Instead, she volunteered at a temporary hospital in Washington, D.C.

In 1862, she also organized a women's relief organization to help families of the wounded. Undaunted by danger, Mary didn't hesitate to step up to the Union front lines, including the Battles of Bull Run and Chickamauga, and even fearlessly crossed Confederate lines to treat civilians. In that same year, Mary moved on to Virginia, treating wounded soldiers throughout the state.

The year 1863 proved to be a milestone for Mary: at long last her medical credentials were finally accepted. She moved to Tennessee, where she was appointed a War Department surgeon with a paid position and rank of captain. Her good deeds didn't escape the dangers of war. She was captured in April 1864 by the South and held as a prisoner of war for four months.

Eventually, she and some other Union doctors were traded in a prisoner-of-war exchange for Confederate medical officers. Rumors remain that she was captured on purpose so she could spy for the North, but they were never proven.

Soon after her release, Mary packed up her doctor's bag to become an assigned medical director at a hospital for women imprisoned in Kentucky.

In 1865, Mary left government service for good and was awarded the Medal of Honor by President Andrew Johnson. It was the high point of her career—and also the lowest. She was the only woman out of 3,500 who received the mark of distinction. What should have been a tribute given in recognition of her dedication to medicine was unfortunately tainted by a controversy. Not only were Mary's manner and way of life brought into question, but a key undermining factor was the fact that Mary was a civilian and had never received an official military commission during the war as well.

Her civilian status is why Mary's medal was rescinded in 1917 along with 910 others. But being the staunch individual that she was, Mary refused to return the medal and continued to wear it the rest of her life. Sixty years later, in 1977, President Jimmy Carter restored the honor in her name, thanks to efforts from her family. Justice was finally served.

Mary died in 1919, the only woman to win the Medal of Honor. She was acclaimed for her patriotism and for being referred to as "that shocking female surgeon in trousers." True to her nature and beliefs, she was buried in a man's suit.

PART 11

IMAGES

SARAH HOPKINS BRADFORD
(1818–1912), "MOSES BIOGRAPHER"

Geneva and Auburn

In today's culture, a white person being friends with a Black person would not raise an eyebrow. However, in the late 1800s, a relationship between an educated white woman and a formerly enslaved Black woman was highly unusual, even scandalous, but these two left a significant mark in history.

Sarah Hopkins Bradford (1818–1912) and Harriet Tubman (1822–1913) were only four years apart in age, yet their circumstances couldn't be further apart. Harriet Tubman is credited with being the leader of seventy freedom seekers who crossed over state lines. (The exact number varies from fifty into the hundreds.) Harriet's name is synonymous with the Underground Railroad; she was fittingly known far and wide as the "Conductor." The history of antislavery that is taught in schools today is due to Harriet and the risks she took for her beliefs in freedom.

She was born into slavery on a plantation in Maryland, where she was overworked and whipped. In 1849, she escaped to Philadelphia and got a job in a hotel. But she had another far more important job as a conductor on the Underground Railroad, a secret route of "stations" for the enslaved heading to the north and Canada. Harriet made nineteen trips back to Maryland, helping her own family gain freedom in 1857. A $40,000 reward for her capture didn't deter her efforts. Harriet and her groups traveled only at night to avoid being seen; if they were caught, it would have meant death. She carried a gun as a threat, but she never used it.

So much has been written about Harriet Tubman that the person who wrote the definitive biography of her becomes overshadowed. Sarah

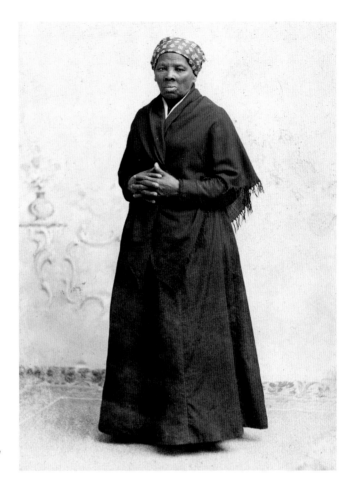

Harriet Tubman.
*Courtesy of the Library
of Congress.*

Hopkins Bradford wrote a definitive two-volume biography of Harriet. What is remarkable about the book, is that as Harriet was enslaved, she couldn't read or write. It was, in fact, illegal, making capturing her story a challenge for Sarah, who had to put pieces of spoken interviews together. An author can't write about Sarah without also including Harriet.

One question regarding the relationship of these two women is how they met. The key factor was the Auburn Central Presbyterian Church Harriet's parents attended. The New York church broke away from the Second Presbyterian Church over the issue of abolition.

Sarah's brother, the Reverend Dr. Samuel Hopkins, was instrumental in the founding of the new church that would become central in their lives. Sarah taught Harriet's parents there, and later, Harriet would be married there.

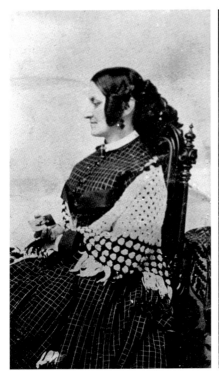 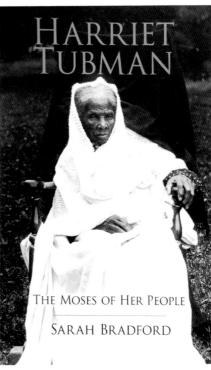

Left: Sarah Hopkins Bradford. *Courtesy of the Geneva Historical Society.*

Right: Cover of Bradford's seminal work. *Author's collection.*

As with most formerly enslaved people, money was an issue, but Harriet was fortunate, as she was able to purchase a house for her family with a loan of $1,200 from Senator William Henry Steward (who would become Lincoln's secretary of state in 1861).

Sarah met Harriet's parents in a Sunday School class when she was visiting her brother in Auburn, New York, during the Civil War. She and her friends decided to publish Harriet's life story as a fundraiser for the church.

Even though she had written two adult biographies of Peter the Great and Christopher Columbus, Sarah was best known as an author of children's books. They were moralistic and didactic, much like Sunday School lessons reflecting the tenor of the times. They were not meant for enjoyment but offered purposeful moral instruction.

Her most successful series was a six-volume set titled the *Silver Lake Series*. Even though the books were a series, each one could stand alone as a collection of poems and short stories. Sarah's first story, "Amy, the Glass

Blower's Daughter," was published in 1847. Included in the series were: *The Budget, The Jumble, Ups and Downs, Green Satchel, The Cornucopia* and *Aunt Patty's Mirror*.

The poet Lydia Maria Child, who was best known for her poem "Over the River and Through the Woods," met Harriet at a Civil War Union camp in Hampton, Virginia. The two women were volunteering to help "contraband," people who had escaped from slavery. Lydia wrote down some of Harriet's words from working together in the camp and also wrote the preface to Sarah's book and edited it. The title of the second edition expresses the role and significance of Harriet Tubman: *Moses of Her People*. Several versions of the book are still available today.

The proceeds from the second book, published in 1886, went to the Harriet Tubman Home for the Aged in Auburn and probably saved Harriet from losing her house.

Meanwhile, Sarah was in grim need for revenue from her own book sales, as her husband had abandoned her and their six children in 1857 to open a law practice in Chicago. She wrote under a pen name of Cousin Cicely.

When her husband died, Sarah opened Mrs. Bradford's School for Young Ladies, where she taught lessons in English and math. Shortly after the publication of the second edition of Harriet's biography, Sarah closed her school and spent eight years traveling around Europe with her daughters. She returned to Rochester, where she died on June 25, 1912, and is buried in the Washington Street Cemetery in Geneva, New York.

Harriet believed that God had commanded her to help free the enslaved, and she applied that faith to help Black soldiers during the Civil War by serving as a nurse, cook and even a spy.

In the annals of women's history, the lives of Sarah and Harriet are intertwined, yet each one left footprints on different paths. They were proud and strong women who were symbiotic friends.

LOUISE BLANCHARD BETHUNE
(1856–1913), "BUILDING CHARACTER"

Waterloo

In the late 1800s, when the only acceptable career choices for women were either teaching or nursing, Jennie Louise Blanchard would change that and prove naysayers wrong: she became the first female architect in America.

As a child, Louise was in poor health, so her parents homeschooled her until she was eleven. Under the tutelage of her father, who was a math teacher and school principal at Waterloo Union School, New York, and her mother, who was a schoolteacher, she was well educated.

When she was in high school in Buffalo, New York, she became known as "Lulu" to her fellow classmates, but it was a daunting remark from a male student who boasted that "girls can't be architects" that crystalized her identity. Instead of intimidating her, his challenge just confirmed her passion for architecture, a field that had not previously been open to women. Louise graduated in 1874, realizing that she would need to call on her strength of character to overcome many obstacles that would stand in her way.

After high school, she spent two years preparing to attend the newly established architecture program at Cornell University. There was just one catch; they didn't accept women. Instead, she studied and traveled, and in 1876, she accepted a position as a draftsman in the office of Richard Waite, a prominent architecture firm in Buffalo, New York. The position was low-paying, but the reason she accepted it was that it gave her access to the business library. For five years, she worked on improving her skills, giving up her plans to study architecture in college but not giving up her penchant for designing buildings.

She then felt ready to open her own business in Buffalo, which she did. The year 1881 was a momentous one for Louise. At age twenty-five, she opened her own private practice with Robert Bethune, making her the first female architect in America. In December of that year, she married Robert, and the company became Bethune & Bethune.

Due to the opening of the Erie Canal, Buffalo was in the eye of an economic boom. The call for high-caliber buildings created a demand for architects, and Louise and her husband were at the right place at the right time. There was ample work for their firm, and in 1890, architect William Fuchs joined them, making Bethune, Bethune & Fuchs the preeminent architectural firm in Buffalo and western New York.

Prior to that, she applied for membership in the Western Association of Architects (WAA) in 1885 and was enthusiastically and unanimously approved by the board of directors. Their action set a precedent for admitting women.

A rare opportunity opened up for Louise when the Women's Building of the World's Columbian Exposition in Chicago in 1893 held a design competition. The perception was that winning the commission would catapult the winner's career into fame. However, Louise refused to enter because she was opposed to competitions in general, but she was incensed when she learned that the winning fee for women was $1,000 while the prize for men was $10,000, implying that women were inferior.

Louise was caught between being a businesswoman and her principles. She didn't want to appear as an antagonizing suffragette, but she also believed in equal pay for equal work. One of her ways of staying abreast of the status of women in the profession was by consistently supporting the New York State Legislature's Architects Licensing Bill, which enforced professional exams to practice architecture.

She also became active in architectural organizations, helping organize the Buffalo Society of Architects and serving as the vice president and treasurer of the Buffalo chapter. Louise was rising to the top floor. In 1888, she was the first woman elected to the American Institute of Architects (AIA), and the next year, she became the AIA's first female fellow.

Though the Bethune firm designed all types of buildings, from industrial to residential, Louise was partial to schools. Starting in 1881, the Buffalo Public Schools District undertook an elaborate plan to build progressive schools that considered the needs of children, and Louise's firm won the contract. All in all, the Bethunes designed eighteen schools while they were in practice.

Louise was a realist, as expressed by this quote from her: "You can't predict the future. It turns out you can't predict the past either. Time moves in both directions—forward and backward—and what happens here and now changes them both." And make changes she did.

Her success reflected her ability to apply new developments in sanitation, fireproofing and ventilation. Her eye for design and innovative approach to construction made her the top architect in Buffalo.

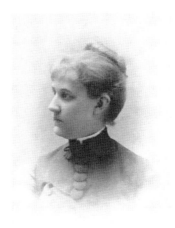

Louise Bethune. *Courtesy of Wikimedia Commons.*

An article about Louise sums up her feelings: "To most people, buildings are simple, cold structures but to Louise, they had feelings with sentiments attached to them."

Of all of the spectacular and functional buildings that Louise designed, one in particular stood out and was her favorite. The Lafayette Hotel in downtown Buffalo was her best-known design and one that would make her famous. Louise commissioned it for $1 million. The result was a seven-story, 225-room Renaissance Revival hotel that featured hot and cold water in all bathrooms as well as telephones. The building was completed in 1904. In today's world of convenience gadgets, the simple amenities back then seemed grandiose. The Lafayette is still in business today and often used for weddings.

During her thirty-year career, Louise made many accomplishments. This quote from the *Buffalo Spree* (Summer 1986) sums up her work: "Not only is it possible for a woman to design buildings, she showed the world that a woman could design great, useful buildings as well as any man."

CLARA WOLCOTT DRISCOLL (1861–1944), "CRACKING THE GLASS CEILING"

Canandaigua

The adage "Behind every successful man is a woman" couldn't be more fitting or crystal-clear for Clara Wolcott Driscoll. Trapped by archaic laws that put married women at a disadvantage, she managed to rise above them and pursue an artistic career.

Born in Tallmadge, Ohio, in 1861, she had three sisters: Kate, Emily and Josephine. The bond between them would be a constant in their lives.

Education was important to the family. Her father, Elizer Wolcott, was a Yale graduate, but it was her mother, Fannie Pierce, who wanted her daughters to be educated. Since Clara showed an aptitude for art, Fannie sent her to design school in Cleveland, where she studied architectural design. After working for a local furniture maker, she moved to New York City and enrolled in the new Metropolitan Museum Art School. That experience and skills led her to Tiffany's Glass Studios.

The reality of the name on the Tiffany artwork belonged to Clara, not Louis Comfort Tiffany. When she won a Bronze Medal at the 1900 Paris World Fair for her signature piece, the dragonfly lamp, the honor exposed that the credit for the elegant creations and intricate handwork belonged to Clara, not Tiffany himself. Even more important was the attention that it brought to her work.

Due to an inequitable law at that time, married women were not allowed to work. Clara managed to maneuver her times around the law and worked at Tiffany on and off for the next twenty years. Her professional life was intertwined with her personal life. She married Francis Driscoll in 1889 at age twenty-seven and quit working. Throughout her life, Clara would be lucky in romance but not marriage. When Francis died three years later, she went back to work. A few years after that, another man entered her life, Edwin Waldo.

She accepted a second wedding engagement and took Edwin home to meet her family in Ohio, but evidently, he got cold feet and disappeared on the trip there. This happened in 1897, and it was believed that Edwin was dead until five years later, when Clara received word via a Cleveland newspaper that Edwin was alive in San Francisco. Instead of bemoaning her situation, Clara went back to work.

She married for the third and, hopefully lucky, last time. She met Edward Booth, an Englishman, who lived in the same boardinghouse as her for ten years. At first, they were friends; then love bloomed, and the couple married in 1907. Their marriage lasted thirty-five years.

Much of the personal life of Clara and her two sisters was detailed in round-robin letters that they wrote. In those days, the letters were a fashionable way of keeping in touch. Each sister would add to the letter and pass it on to the next, keeping the circle going, as the name suggests.

After Emily died, a treasure of 1,163 round-robin letters was found in a summer cabin near Canandaigua Lake. Those letters are now housed in the Kent State University Library (Ohio) and the Queens Historical Society. Without those letters, Clara and her achievements would have been virtually unknown.

An article in the *Daily News* in 1904 described Clara by saying: "This is rather difficult work [referring to glass designing and cutting] but when one has a fondness for a certain brand of industry, she does not pause when a difficulty must be overcome. The work is a new departure for women and I believe they like it."

The Tiffany Glass Studio closed in 1932, and Clara died in 1944 at the age of eighty-two. Ironically, her death certificate listed her as "occupation housewife."

In 1888 she was one of a few women who made $10,000 a year. She went from earning $20 a week when she started at Tiffany's to creating beautiful artwork worth thousands and more. However, in spite of her income, Clara couldn't afford to buy one of her own

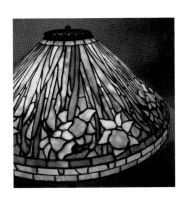

Tiffany Studios Daffodil glass table lamp designed by Driscoll. *Courtesy of Wikimedia Commons.*

lamps. In the late 1800s, Tiffany lamps cost anywhere from $250 to $400. In today's world, an original Tiffany lamp was sold at a Christie's auction in 1998 for $2.8 million.

While many of Clara's contributions were anonymous, she was the guiding light behind Tiffany's success in crafting beautiful glasswork. In a *New York Times* article on February 26, 2007, Jeffrey Kastner described Clara as "a hidden creative force behind a legendary object in the history of American arts; the Tiffany lamp." And she was. Clara broke the glass ceiling, and her work continues to make headlines today with traveling exhibitions and published books, even novels.

MAUD HUMPHREY
(1868–1940), "PICTURE PERFECT"

Canandaigua

Here's looking at you, kid! This infamous line of dialogue was said in 1942 in a film titled *Casablanca* by a young male actor. While many mothers could brag that their sons were doctors or lawyers, only Maud Humphrey could boast that her son was the famous movie star, Bogie.

Maud was a popular painter of cherubic children who spent her summers on Canandaigua Lake. However, she had another claim to fame: her artwork. Mother and son each left memorable impressions in their worlds of art and acting.

Maud was born in 1868 in Rochester, New York, in an area known as the Ruffled Shirt district (now known as Corn Hill) to a prominent family. She displayed an early talent for art, taking evening art classes at the age of twelve. By her late teens, she had landed her first commissions for black-and-white illustrations.

By the mid-1800s, she had moved to New York City and entered the new Arts Students League and won a Louis Prang and Company Christmas Card design. Next she began working for Frederick A. Stokes as a book illustrator. Maud was on her way.

From there it was off to Paris to study at the Académie Julian, where she trained under the famed James McNeill Whistler. By 1893, Maud had found her niche—painting adorable children—and by the turn of the century, she had become one of the best and most successful commercial illustrators.

In fact, Maud made more money than her husband, which was highly unusual at the time. Reports claimed Maud earned over $50,000 a year

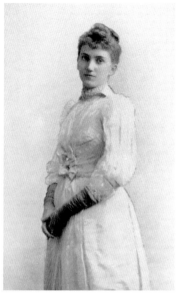 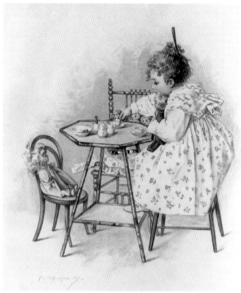

Left: Portrait of Maud Humphrey. *Courtesy of Wikimedia Commons.*

Right: Humphrey illustration, "Maternal Cares." *Courtesy of the Library of Congress.*

to her husband's $20,000 as a heart surgeon. It was a bone of contention between them and still an issue for some couples today.

Maud's technique of using dry watercolors was a perfect medium for portraying adorable children in active scenes instead of prim, posed portraits. Her style quickly became popular. Her angelic faces were ideal for ad campaigns such as Ivory soap, Mullins baby food and Crosman Brothers flower seeds, all featuring her winsome images.

Maud often used real children for models, but despite rumors, her son, Bogie, was not the model for the Gerber food label, though he was cute enough. Many of the young girls she painted were adorable, with rosy cheeks, red lips and curly blond ringlets, and wore starched dresses with frilly collars.

In the summer of 1899, Dr. Belmont Deforest Bogart bought fifty-five acres of ground on Canandaigua Lake for his pregnant wife. The estate was named Willow Brook. Bogie arrived on Christmas Day, one year after his parents' marriage in 1898. Two sisters followed, and Willow Brook became a summertime haven for the three children to escape the turmoil at home.

By 1910, the Humphreys were well-off enough financially that they could afford a four-story townhouse on West 103rd Street in New York City. Maud's husband was a cardio-pulmonary specialist and saw patients on the first floor. Maud worked in a studio on the fourth floor, and they shared the rest of the space with their servants.

Her studio was as immaculate as her smocks and aprons. She painted standing up, dressed in shades of gray with white and pink accents. Scarves, bows and ribbons completed her outfits. She was tall, five feet, ten inches, and always wore high-heeled shoes, even when painting. In contrast, her shoe size was just two and a half.

Maud treated her children with a combination of indifference and criticism. Bogie's childhood was stifling, caught between his parents' careers. He was small in stature with a sissy name and dressed in fussy clothes by his mother—a perfect target for teasing. His father would often explode in anger, disciplining the children with a belt.

On the outside, the household was the epitome of gracious Victorian living, while the inside of the house was filled with anger and abuse. No wonder the kids escaped to Willow Brook for the summers.

Both parents were in poor health. Belmont was in chronic pain from a carriage accident. Year by year, he sank further into morphine addiction. Maud had migraines and a painful bacterial skin condition. She also abused alcohol. Sadly, they both became addicted to morphine.

At the peak of her career, when Maud was a household name, she turned to a more sophisticated style of illustration—fashion. In the late 1900s, she became the art director for *The Delineation* magazine. It was the perfect venue for her art. Sewing pattern companies and other women's magazines were eager to display her paintings. She was most proud of this position because it published articles about her favorite cause, women's suffrage.

Like other fashionable families, the Bogarts' summer cottage was a haven for sailing and other activities until 1915, when they sold the property for another summer home on Fire Island, New York. The move enabled Maud to work closer to home.

Then the Depression hit (1929–39), and the family fortune disappeared. Belmont died, and Maud was left with thousands of dollars in hospital debt. Her son came to her rescue and paid off the debt and moved his mother to California. Living in a studio apartment on Sunset Boulevard was quite a change in lifestyle for Maud, but her creativity continued to bloom as she applied her artistic talent to greeting cards, calendars and books.

Among the twenty-some books that she illustrated were: *Mother Goose, Babes of the Year* and *Sleepy Times Stories*. Any of her paintings, whether on greeting cards, calendars or magazines, are considered highly collectible today.

After five years of retirement, Maud died of pneumonia and cancer on November 22, 1940, and is buried in Forest Lawn Cemetery in Los Angeles. Ironically, her death certificate lists her as "housewife"—certainly an inadequate term for Maud. Both mother and son left indelible marks in art and film.

PEARL WHITE
(1889–1938), "SILENT FILMS"

Ithaca

Outside the theater, the marquee flashed bright lights with the name of the film starring Pearl White. Inside the theater, the seats were filled with people eagerly awaiting the latest thriller and cliffhanger movie. Who was this young actress from Missouri, and how did she become a major player of worldwide fame?

Today, few people will recognize her name unless they are fans of early silent films, but in her day in the 1920s, Pearl was the queen of serial films, as famous as Charlie Chaplin and Mary Pickford.

Born in 1889 in Missouri, Pearl had a childhood that was far from normal. She toured with her parents in stock companies throughout the American Midwest. A primary source of entertainment at that time was dramatic shows, and Pearl made her stage debut at the age of six playing Little Eva in *Uncle Tom's Cabin*. Her next performances were from 1902 to 1909, when she worked as a bareback rider in the circus until she suffered a riding injury. Did that deter Pearl from performing on horses? Of course not—she was a performer at heart. She simply switched to acting in over one hundred western two-reelers and starring in *The Life of Buffalo Bill*.

Her breakthrough year was 1910, when she made her debut in films. Her popularity crossed the ocean and came to the attention of Pathé Frères, the major French film company. It was producing its first American film, *The Girl from Arizona*, in a new studio in New Jersey, and Pearl was the perfect choice for the heroine. That little girl from Missouri was hitting the big time. Other film companies also gave her top billing in a number of slapstick comedy shorts. Her popularity was growing.

Pathé director Louis Gasnier offered her the starring role in a film serial *The Perils of Pauline* featuring the central character of "Pauline." Her popularity was growing with each chapter. In 1914 and 1915, she was the most popular female star in silent films, even topping Mary Pickford at the box office.

Whether flying airplanes, racing cars or swimming across rivers, Pearl did most of her own stunt work for publicity purposes. For one of those thrillers, she dangled from a tall Manhattan building just to paint her

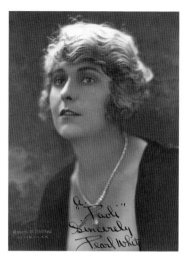

Pearl White. *Courtesy of Wikimedia Commons.*

initials on the brick wall. A headline in *American Magazine* dated September 1921 called her "the heroine of a thousand dangerous stunts." The dangers in the films were real, and when the hazardous acts began to cause serious injuries, she was forced to use stunt doubles.

Pearl relied on alcohol to numb her constant pain and ended up being hospitalized in 1933 for addiction. Sadly, she became more addicted to the drugs used during her treatment. She was quoted as saying; "I have actually gotten used to the fear."

Between 1912 and 1920, Ithaca was the center of silent films. The location of gorges and waterfalls around Cayuga Lake was perfect for scenic backgrounds while the locals were dazzled by her antics.

Pearl bought a canary yellow convertible Sutz Bearcat and loved zooming around town in her flashy car. In 1919, a Stutz Bearcat cost $3,250 (the equivalent today would be around $50,000 and up to $1 million). Her salary in the beginning was $250 per week. That amount rose as quickly as her fame. Pearl was wealthy!

One version of how she loved playing to the crowd was when she raced through town and was given a ticket, which she promptly tore up. To say she was flamboyant would be an understatement. As an attractive, buxom blond, she drew lots of attention. If she wanted to go out and be unnoticed, she simply took off her blond hair, revealing that it was a wig. Her own hair was her disguise.

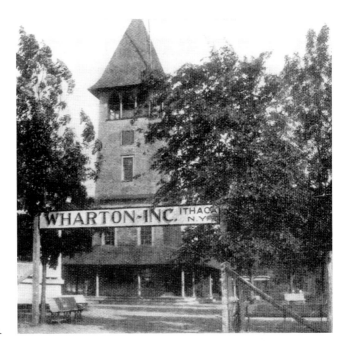

Wharton Studio in Ithaca. *Courtesy of the Wharton Studio Museum.*

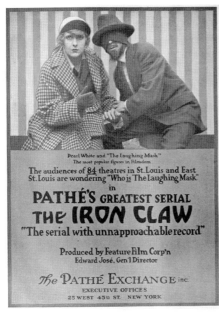

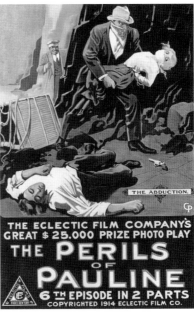

Left: Advertisement for Pathé's *The Iron Claw*, starring Pearl White. *Courtesy of Wikimedia Commons.*

Right: Movie poster for *The Perils of Pauline*, starring Pearl White. *Courtesy of Wikimedia Commons.*

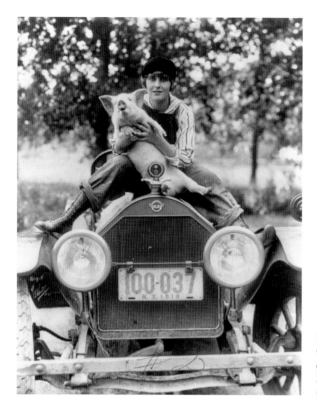

Pearl White holding a pig
while seated on the hood
of a Stutz automobile with
New York license plate.
Courtesy of Library of Congress.

Her good looks naturally drew the attention off many men, and Pearl was married twice. The first was an actor, Victor Sutherland, whom she met while performing with the Trousdale Stock Company, a traveling acting troupe. That marriage ended in divorce in 1914. Her second husband, Wallace McCutcheon Jr., was also an actor and a World War I vet who suffered mental problems from being gassed. That marriage didn't last either. They divorced in 1921, and he eventually died by suicide.

What caused the film industry to move to Hollywood was the severity of Finger Lakes weather, which wasn't conducive to year-round filmmaking, so the industry moved west to a warmer climate.

Due to Pathé's international distribution unit, Pearl's films were shown in many countries abroad. She now had an international reputation, and heaps of fan mail arrived from all over the world.

All in all, Pearl made over two hundred films. The most popular ones were the cliffhanger series. Without today's venues of modern amusement, the major form of public amusement was the black-and-white melodramas. Audiences were eager to see Pearl as the "damsel in distress." Each serial had

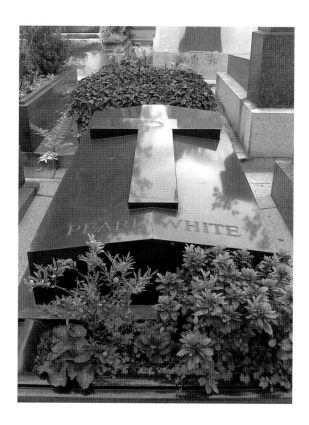

Pearl White grave in Passy, Paris, France. *Courtesy of Wikimedia Commons.*

twenty episodes, lasting six to ten minutes, just enough to tease the audience to come back for the next installment.

The premier of *The Perils of Pauline* was March 31, 1914, at the Loew's Broadway Theatre in Manhattan. Six more serials followed the first with Pearl performing breathtaking stunts:

1914: *Exploits of Pauline*
1915: *New Exploits of Pauline*
1916: *Iron Claw*
1919: *Lightning Raider*
1919: *Black Secret*
1923: *Plunder*

Pearl was born into poverty but became a shrewd businesswoman. When she failed to transition to making feature films because her voice was deemed unsuitable and her health was deteriorating, she retired in 1920 and in 1923 moved to France. By then, she had earned close to $2 million and invested it wisely in a Parisian nightclub, a hotel casino and a stable of profitable racehorses.

She enjoyed a life of luxury until 1937, when the pain and her drug abuse increased from the injuries she suffered in the making of *The Perils of Pauline*. She checked herself into the American Hospital of Paris in July 1938, where she slipped into a coma and died on August 4 due to liver failure. She is buried in Paris.

It was a bit of irony that Paramount released a movie about Pearl the movie star in 1947. The film was a satire on Pearl's rise to fame. It was titled *The Perils of Pauline* and starred Betty Hutton as Pearl. Unfortunately, Pearl died before it opened, negating her opinion on the performance.

For all that Pearl contributed to the history of movies, including a star on the Hollywood Walk of Fame, her tombstone simply states her name: Pearl White.

ELOISE MARGARET WILKIN
(1904–1987), "GOLDEN LEGACY"

Canandaigua

The year was 1946: the Nuremberg trials were held in Tokyo, bikinis went on sale in Paris, the United Nations held its first meeting and the age of baby boomers began. Two years earlier, a little-known artist made an impact on children's book illustration that would last for decades.

Eloise Wilkin was just eleven when she won a drawing contest, which was the beginning of a charmed career. After completing a college course in illustration at the Rochester Institute of Technology in 1923, she and her friend Joan Esley opened an art gallery in Rochester, New York. Unfortunately, the studio was unsuccessful, but Eloise was undaunted.

She moved to New York City and did freelance work for many publishing companies. In 1927, Century Company is credited with giving Eloise her first book to illustrate, *The Shining Hours*. And shine she did. Eloise was on her way to a golden career.

Three subjects were prevalent throughout her art: nature and the outdoors, religion and family life. She often illustrated religious picture books that included compilations of prayers. Now and then, she painted some titles that were written by her sister, children's author Ester Burns Wilkin.

In 1935, she married Stanley Wilkin, and Eloise cut back on her illustrating to raise four children. During that time, she used family members and neighbors as models. Her medium was watercolors with soft colored pencil lines to delicately create adorable, chubby-cheeked children that became her signature.

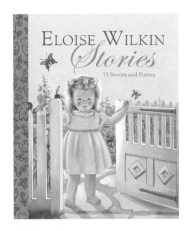

A Wilkin Little Golden Book.
Author's collection.

Little Golden books were launched in 1942 with twelve titles, each priced at twenty-five cents, and sold where women shopped. Instead of the usual print run of five thousand copies, twenty-five thousand copies each were printed, proving that the affordable cost and the smart merchandising would attract sales, which they did big-time. They were an instant sensation, catapulting them to the top of popularity, selling thousands of the books.

Her vintage background scenes detail early American and Victorian furnishings, down to the architecture and wallpaper. The landscapes that she drew were drawn from the areas she frequented, family gatherings and summers in Canandaigua. In *Happy Birthday*, the child in pigtails was her granddaughter. As an example of how precise her work was, the father in *Help Daddy* was Eloise's husband, and she painted him as left-handed when he was right-handed. The publisher asked her to change it, and she did.

While her work was always meticulous, keen eyes may notice one missing detail. She never drew children with their teeth showing, just closed-mouth smiles. Evidently, she wasn't satisfied with how they looked.

Throughout her vocation, Eloise was attuned to cultural changes. The 1954 cover of *The New Baby* pictures a baby sleeping on her tummy. The image was changed due to public awareness of sudden death syndrome at that time.

The original 1956 edition of *My Little Golden Book* about God featured white children only. Eloise was ahead of the times, before diversity became a societal focus. Being sensitive to racial portrayals, she re-illustrated several pages to include children of other races.

In 1982, Little Golden Books turned forty, and over 800 million copies had been sold. On November 20, 1986, 1 billion books were sold, and the all-time favorite, *The Pokey Little Puppy*, was printed. The book's popularity spread to every country in the world, except for the Soviet Union, which considered it too capitalistic. Few children's books have had the staying power of the *Puppy*, as it has never been out of print.

Like many young girls her age, Eloise loved to play with dolls, which, no doubt, accounted for her love of baby dolls. She strongly disapproved of the suggestive figures like Barbie that were being merchandised. Instead, she spent years sculpting and perfecting clay models of baby doll heads. It took until 1959 for her to be satisfied that she had created the most realistic head to take to Vogue Dolls. The doll manufacturer immediately launched the first doll designed by Eloise. Baby Dear was "born" and became an overnight sensation. In all, Eloise designed eight dolls for Vogue and Madame Alexander Dolls, another popular and collectible doll.

F.A.O. Schwartz, the famous toy store in New York City, featured a whole window display of Baby Dear. At the same time, the United Nations was in session; the infamous Russian ruler Nikita Khrushchev was so charmed with the doll that he and his delegation bought thirteen of them to take back to Russia. Never mind capitalism. The first Christmas that Baby Dear was on the market, it sold over 100,000 units. The appeal of the doll was how realistic it looked, with a vinyl head and cloth body. It even had a small section of hair rooted to the crown.

All in all, Eloise illustrated forty-seven Golden books, eight dolls and assorted puzzles, greeting cards and posters, even china plates. Her imprint was everywhere. Anything she painted is highly collectible.

For people familiar with children's books, they will be amused by a different Eloise, a doll dressed as Eloise from the book about the irrepressible little girl who lives in the Plaza Hotel in New York City, written by Hilary Knight. One wonders what Eloise the illustrator thought.

Golden books have become classics with devoted collectors. A first edition with a blue spine can bring as much as $800 or higher, depending on condition, edition and age. In the 1960s, the price increased from

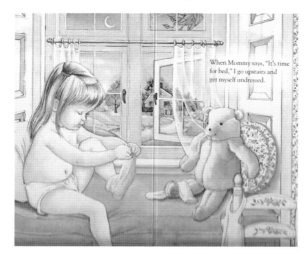

My Goodnight Book, 1981.
Author's collection.

53

the original $0.25 to $0.29 and the blue spine was changed to antique gold. There are two important books about Eloise and Golden Books that provide more insight into her artistic talent and place in children's book illustration.

The title of the first one is explanatory: *How Golden Books Won Children's Hearts, Changed Publishing Forever and Became an American Icon Along the Way*. The book was published by Golden Books/Random Books in 2007 and was written by children's book historian Leonard Marcus.

The other book is more personal. *The Golden Years of Eloise Wilkin* was intended to be a joint effort with daughter Deborah Wilkin Springett and her mother. But poor health intervened. Eloise died before her daughter could tell her story. Instead, the book became a dual narrative; the top half of the page was a straightforward account of Eloise's life; the bottom half was a separate accounting in script font recalling family memories written by Deborah from her childhood.

During her career, Eloise illustrated more than one hundred books and created many dolls. Her golden legacy touched millions of adults and families and, most significantly, helped instill a love of reading in children.

Eloise died from cancer at age eighty-three and is buried in the Holy Sepulcher Cemetery in Rochester.

ELOISE THEODORA WOOD
(1897–1966), "ETCHER"

Geneva

Is it pure coincidence that two women in the early 1900s had the same first name, outstanding careers in art and deep roots to the Finger lakes? Most likely. Though their lives overlapped, research could not verify that they knew each other. So, Eloise Wood (1897–1966), meet Eloise Wilkin (1904–1987). Both artists were accomplished with signature styles—Wood for her engravings and Wilkin for her cherubic children.

Eloise Wood was born in 1897 to John and Mary Sill Wood, while Eloise Wilkin was born in 1904, a third-generation Genevan with strong ties to the Finger Lakes. While their life spans overlapped, each chose different art techniques. Wood's mother recognized her daughter's talent early in her childhood and kept a scrapbook filled with her drawings and photos of her many performances.

Her education began by attending schools in Geneva, with a brief stint at William Smith College in Geneva. Eloise rounded up her studies in Buffalo, New York, where she transferred to the highly regarded Albright Art School in 1915, finishing her degree there. But the big city called her, and she moved to New York City, teaching at several art schools and attending Columbia University's Teachers College.

She lived through both world wars and joined the Ambulance Corps in World War I at age nineteen. After living in New York City during the late 1920s and early '30s, she returned to Geneva to care for aging family members. That block of time allowed her to cultivate her art, especially her focus and interest in etching. Whether it was her meticulous nature or patriotic duty, Wood joined a handful of women who enrolled in courses at the Geneva School of Automobile Engineers.

Art wasn't her only gift. She continued to hone her talents in singing, performing, even writing plays. She appeared many times in concerts and plays put on by the Geneva Woman's Club. One in particular, she wrote specifically for the Geneva City Hospital as a fundraiser, called *Your Ox or Mine: A Comedy of Greenwich Village*. It was performed at the Smith Opera House in Geneva in 1924, mocking the Village's bohemian lifestyle and displaying her sense of humor. The proceeds went to a contagious unit.

Eloise transferred her skills to teaching and was the only art instructor for Hobart and William Smith Colleges, replacing Norman Kent (1903–1972), who had pioneered the position, but she developed her own courses for the art departments. Both Kent and Wood were featured in an exhibition at the Geneva History Museum in 1971—Kent for his woodcuts and Wood for her engravings.

In World War II, she began working for the American Can Company in its camouflage and drafting departments, though it seemed like an odd job move at the time, as the company manufactured tin cans. However, when her drawing skills were recognized, she was recruited to teach mechanical drawing at Hobart and Smith Colleges in Geneva for the V-12 and V-5 military units stationed there.

By 1947, Wood had not only mastered but also taught almost every medium and style of painting and drawing—from charcoal to European-style oils. Displays of her work were not limited to local areas. She exhibited her work at the Brooklyn Society of Etchers and hosted several one-woman shows. She even sold an etching (*Lilies*) to the Metropolitan Museum of Art.

The process of etching requires precision and a steady hand. It involves creating a picture on a metal plate by using acid to eat away unwanted lines and indentations. The empty spaces are then filled with ink or wax, making a smooth surface for the artist to scratch an image with a sharp needle. The difference between etching and engraving is etching uses acid to burn lines into metal while engraving is created by using sharp tools. Wood used both.

Wood's range of artwork was impressive, from florals, animals and buildings to large-scale art projects, such as stained-glass windows at an area chapel. Other creations included forty-one heraldic plaques for the

Coxe Auditorium, named for Hobart College's benefactor, and five panels for the Gothic niches at St. John's Chapel in Manhattan.

Throughout her career, her favorite technique was always etching. In 1965, she was awarded a full professorship at the Colleges but sadly died less than a year later at age sixty-eight. Eloise left a legacy and etched her name in art history and more than earned the moniker of "pioneer female artist."

GRACE ADELLE WOODWORTH
(1872–1967), "SMILE!"

Seneca Falls

G race Woodworth was growing up during the same period that photography and cameras were developing into a fashionable and fascinating art form.

What drew Grace to photography is sketchy. As she recalled, her parents; younger sister, Edith; an older sister, Jeannie; and one brother, Elmer, all lived a comfortable middle-class life in the small town of Seneca Falls, New York.

She was greatly influenced by her father, Josiah, who was a self-made man with a penchant for learning. (He bragged that he owned eighty-three books.) When she was eight, his dry goods store failed and circumstances changed, making it necessary for him to take two jobs as a traveling agent for two different companies. Instead of blaming him for his failure, like others did, Grace chose to admire his willingness to work for others.

Her mother, Edna Miller, was Josiah's second wife. A member of the family described her as a "lady," meaning she didn't work. Edna never approved of Grace's "work" because it wasn't ladylike. That didn't deter Grace; if being frowned at bothered her, she didn't show it.

She attended Seneca Falls' public high school, where she was described as a "restless adventurous spirit," probably because she loved to read, dance and paint, choosing to venture outside the expected role of women of the times. She wanted to be considered an individualist, not a feminist, making a distinction between the two characterizations.

She was definitely an independent woman. She graduated in 1890 and, by choice, never married, as was true of her older sister, Jeannie. Both chose

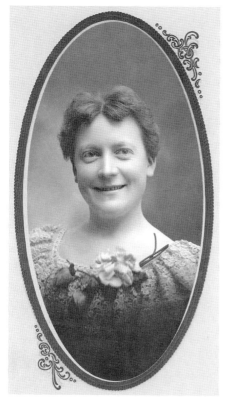

Left: Grace Woodworth. *Courtesy of the Seneca Falls Historical Society.*

Below: The Woodworths. *Courtesy of the Seneca Falls Historical Society.*

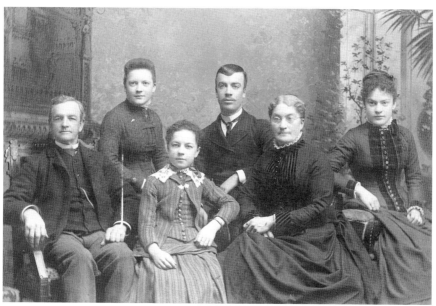

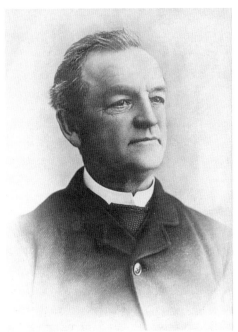
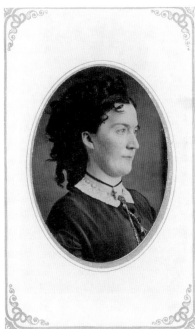

Left: Josiah Woodworth. *Courtesy of the Seneca Falls Historical Society.*

Right: Edna Miller Woodworth. *Courtesy of the Seneca Falls Historical Society.*

to forego the life of the "ideal" woman as head of a middle-class household and remained single.

The beginning of Grace's awareness of women's issues was initiated by her father's freethinking and convictions; plus the fact that he didn't smoke or drink encouraged Grace to become involved in the Seneca Falls Christian Temperance Union.

At this point, photography entered Grace's life. As Grace had taught herself to paint, an aunt noticed her talent and encouraged her to try photography, which she did. It was a natural fit. Next came a job as a retoucher for a Batavia, New York photographer, and Grace was hooked. She seriously studied the techniques and capabilities of the newest artistic invention. At the encouragement of other photographers, Grace bought her first studio from George H. Richards in Union Springs, New York, near Cayuga Lake.

Though the field of photography was expanding in the 1880s, it was dominated by men. By contrast, Grace was exceptional by gender, business sense, age (twenty-five) and proficiency.

The *Union Springs Advertiser* stated, "Miss Woodworth is a young lady of several years' experience in the photographic business and, in conducting a first-class studio here, gives to the public an opportunity to obtain photos in any of the latest styles or finish, at the lowest prices that first-class work can be made. You are invited to call at the studio and examine work, and also to become acquainted."

She quickly became known as "the lady photographer," as there was little competition from other women. Though she appeared to be prim and proper, there was no question that Grace had the mettle to carry her heavy equipment of a bulky camera, tripod and glass plates when she wanted to take photos of a variety of outdoor scenes. Film cameras would follow much later.

The fact that Grace was a woman in a man's field wasn't a hindrance to her photography business; instead, it proved to be an asset. She enjoyed working with people. As word spread about her flair in making pleasing images of adults, her business soared. Women, in particular, loved having their fancy attire displayed, but it was her photos of children that were exceptional. Instead of having the children pose in a stiff formal position like the adults, she gave them toys to portray them playing in natural surroundings. Filming children became her specialty.

After three years in Union Springs, Grace bought the gallery of Ranger and Whitmore in the Reynolds Arcade in Rochester. The opening announcement invited people to view her work and promised souvenirs. Grace boarded with a Quaker family, which led to the pivotal point in her career. She attended the First Unitarian Church with the family, and it was there she met Susan B. Anthony. The two women took an immediate liking to each other. In spite of their difference in age, they were true kindred spirits.

Grace made many visits to Susan B.'s and Mary's red brick home on Madison Street in Rochester, New York. On one trip, she found Susan's photographic album and knew right away she wanted to take a memorable photo of her revered friend. Grace was commissioned by the Rochester Political Equality Club to take pictures of the sisters for a program celebrating Susan B. on her eighty-fifth birthday in February 1905. When Grace asked Susan B. for permission to have her sit, she was surprised and disappointed when her friend said no, but providence intervened. It was one of their usual conversations about the pursuit of woman's rights that prompted Susan B. to change her mind and agreed to have her photo taken. There were two reasons for her change of heart: one was that Grace was a businesswoman with her own photography studios, and second she

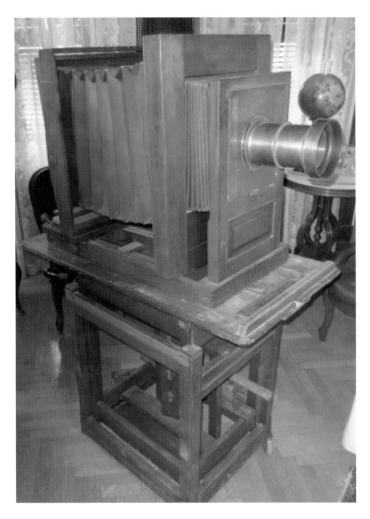

Grace's brass
portrait camera.
Courtesy of the
Seneca Falls
Historical Society.

was from Seneca Falls, the hub of suffragist activity. Both were priorities in the suffragist movement.

As agreed, Susan B. and Mary went to Grace's studio to make the prearranged last photographs of the two of them.

The sisters arrived on time. Susan B. wore a velvet dress with old rose point lace, which she said she had for twenty-two years. Her white hair was parted in the middle and rolled over side combs, and over her shoulder, she wore her well-known little red shawl under her black wrap and her bonnet placed beside her.

When Grace began, Susan B. said, "Now you must make us look very handsome." She took photos of both women, separately and together. But it was when Susan B. thought Grace had exposed the last plate that she relaxed her pose. That image was the one that her friends chose as the official photograph of the famous suffragist: a tired, dignified lady.

It would be her most famous photograph.

In gratitude for the images, Susan B. gave Grace a two-volume edition of her life and inscribed the second volume: "This is given in slight recognition of my pleasure at your success in the art of photography. I rejoice over every young woman who achieves an accomplishment outside the common lines. With the best wishes of your friend, Susan B."

Cameras and photography have made significant advances since Grace's lifetime. The apparatus that was heavy and clumsy has developed into a small hand-held device. Due to the woman known as the "lady photographer" who dared to go "outside the common grounds," Grace Woodworth's photographic profile of Susan B. Anthony left its mark in the annals of women's history by being acclaimed the official imprint and lasting tribute to the woman who spearheaded the women's rights cause.

PART III

INFLUENCERS

AMANDA THEODOSIA JONES (1835–1914), "PRESERVATIONIST"

Bloomfield

To say that Amanda Jones was a remarkable woman would be an understatement. As an inventor, she was awarded two patents: one for food preservation and canning and the other for the use of oil for fuel for furnaces.

She applied her expertise in canning and food preservation by starting her own all-woman business in 1890. Unfortunately, the venture failed.

In many ways, her life was a dichotomy between her literary side and her scientific side. Poetry seemed to be her forte. She had forefathers in both the Revolutionary War and Civil War that provided poetic musings on both.

The average family size in her time was roughly seven children, but Amanda's was an exception. She was one of twelve children (or thirteen depending on the source). The sibling she was closest to was Andrew—or rather his spirit.

In 1859, she contracted tuberculous and endured spending time in compressed air tanks.

For a scientific-minded woman, it seems highly unusual that she was heavily influenced by spiritualism. In 1910, she published *A Psychic Autobiography*, advised by her dead brother, Andrew. She considered herself a medium and relied on her spirits to make decisions, such as moving to Chicago. She relied on his decisions as a guiding force in her life.

Again, following her spirits' advice, she created a second invention: an oil burner, patented in 1880. Again her attempts to turn her inventions into a successful business failed. She said, "This is a women's industry. No man will transact our business, pronounce [*sic*] women's wages or supervise our factories. Give men what ever work is suitable, but keep governing power. Here is a mission, let it be fulfilled." Unfortunately, her words failed her, leaving her significant contributions to her multiple patents and the Jones method for preserving food. She invented processes for safely preserving and canning both wet and dry food and liquids.

It involved steaming sealed jars filled with fruits and vegetables in a light syrup, forcing the air out of the jar and creating an airtight seal. Her patents would benefit home canners and food preservers across the country.

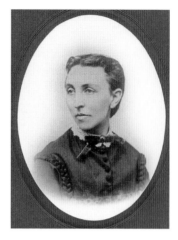

Jones, 1879. *Courtesy of Wikimedia Commons.*

In 1882, she put science behind her, sold her patents and returned to writing, publishing *A Prairie Idyll*. Amanda Jones was indeed a distinctive and remarkable woman. She died of influenza.

AMELIA BLOOMER
(1818–1894), "FASHIONISTA"

Homer

The phrase "put on your big girl pants" is a current idiom that a woman in the 1800s would definitely not comprehend because women simply didn't wear pants! In historic times, women's clothing was cumbersome, restrictive and sometimes just unhealthy. It would take a no-nonsense, determined and practical woman to radically change feminine attire. That woman was Amelia Bloomer. She is credited with launching the term *bloomers* as an alternative for pants.

Amelia was dedicated to working for temperance and women's rights, and bloomers filled the bill. Under her influence, a new fashion was born.

How did a young girl from Homer, New York, wind up being a key figure in the suffrage movement?

Amelia's early years were unremarkable for the times. Occupations for women were limited, mostly as teachers, and she briefly taught school at age seventeen before moving in with her newly married sister living in Waterloo, New York. That too, lasted a short time before she moved into the home of a Seneca Falls family as a live-in governess.

It was there that romance took her on a new path when she married attorney Dexter Bloomer, the owner of the *Seneca Falls County Courier* newspaper. He was so supportive of her involvement in the temperance movement that he gave up drinking.

Temperance was Amelia's primary interest until the Women's Rights Convention in Syracuse, New York, was announced in the *Courier*. It was the first women's rights convention, and Amelia joined and soon became

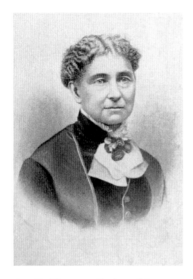

Amelia Bloomer. *Courtesy of the Library of Congress.*

an officer of the Seneca Falls Temperance Society and edited their newspaper. The *Lily* was the first journal for women and was devoted to temperance and other interests of women. Amelia claimed that the paper was the only one owned, edited and published by a woman.

The *Lily* was published from 1849 to 1853 and had a circulation of over four thousand. The contents initially focused on temperance but gradually recipes, education, child-bearing and suffragist tracts began to emerge. However, not everything came up smelling like roses, as there were plenty of obstacles and ridicule from the opposite sex. Despite that, the *Lily* became the model for periodicals focusing on women's suffrage and women's rights.

Scary stories about the effects of alcohol were perpetuated and intended to threaten men who indulged. An example printed in the May 1849 issue cited: "A man when drunk fell into a kettle of boiling brine…and was scaled [scalded] to death."

The year 1851 was pivotal in the crusade for women's rights for two reasons: Amelia introduced Susan B. Anthony to Elizabeth Stanton, the two foremost figures in the suffragist movement, and Amelia was instrumental in starting a fashion revolution.

In the mid-1800s, modesty dictated that American women wear floor-length dresses with a full skirt and waist-pinching corsets and six to eight petticoats underneath. Altogether, the outfit weighed up to fifteen pounds, making breathing difficult.

Wearing bloomers became controversial (mostly perpetuated by men), but in 1853, when she delivered a lecture on the new fashion and women's issues in New York City, three thousand people bought tickets. She had become a national figure.

A fellow suffragette, Libby Smith, had returned from a European trip wearing long, full Turkish trousers under a short skirt that reached just below the knee. Amelia was so taken with the costume that she made one for herself for traveling and promoted the pantaloons with a sketch in the *Lily.*

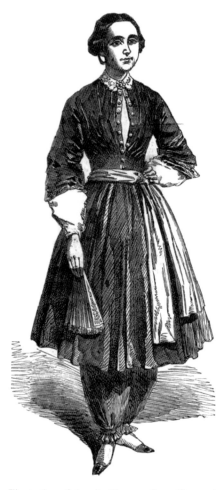

Illustration of Amelia Bloomer from *Illustrated London News. Courtesy of Wikimedia Commons.*

It was no time at all before women everywhere adopted the style and set a trend. Not only were the new pants comfortable, but the knee-length divided trousers made it easier and safer for cycling and other athletic activities as well.

Amelia didn't want the credit for naming the new vogue and felt it should go to Libby Smith, but her protest came too late. Women had already begun to embrace the practicality of the new trend, and with Amelia's promotion of the latest fashion, the term *bloomers* was born. Gone were the waist-pinching girdles and restrictive clothing that hampered every movement. Men jeered and women cheered.

Amelia played a significant hand in the crusade for women's rights all her life, leaving a footprint in its history. In 1995, she was inducted into the National Women's Hall of Fame in Seneca Falls, New York.

In 1999, artist Ted Aub was commissioned to create a statue in honor of the 150th anniversary of the 1848 Women's Rights Convention. It commemorates the contributions of Bloomer, Susan B. Anthony and Elizabeth Stanton, fellow advocates of women's rights. The life-size bronze sculpture depicts the three women with arms interlocked overlooking Van Cleef Lake in Seneca Falls, New York. The title, *When Anthony Met Stanton*, is a reminder and lasting tribute to women who fought for women's rights and continuing the female revolution.

EUNICE NEWTON FOOTE
(1819–1888), "CLIMATOLOGIST"

Bloomfield

In the mid-1800s, scientists were always men—that is, until Eunice Newton Foote broke that barrier. She was a female pioneer in science as well as a botany expert and a women's rights advocate. Her dedication to research was due to her parents. Isaac and Thirza Foote were considered to be a modern couple, especially since they valued education for all of their twelve children, six boys and six girls, but it was Eunice, the youngest, who would make an impact on the field of science and in women's history.

In 1821, the family moved to Bloomfield, New York, where they cultivated a prosperous farm. Eunice continued her education by attending secondary school at the Female Seminary in Troy, New York, where she studied science and botany. It was serendipitous that the seminary had developed a unique program headed by Amos Eaton, a famous American botanist and natural scientist and a supporter of women's rights. He believed that the failure of women in scientific endeavors was not due to a "perversion of the female genus" but due to the lack of opportunity, as female intellect was shockingly equal to that of men.

An example of unfair gender bias occurred in 1856. Eunice had conducted rigorous scientific experiments and written a paper describing the effects of carbon dioxide (CO_2) in trapping atmospheric heat. Unfortunately, women were not allowed to read their own papers, but fortunately for Eunice, distinguished professor Joseph Henry from the Smithsonian Institute read it for her. "Circumstances Affecting the Heat of the Sun's Rays" was proof of Eunice's work.

Without railroads, automobiles or trains, rapid transit in those days was limited to packet boats. These were river steamers on the Erie Canal that were pulled along by horses or mules. Packet boats carried only passengers and their hand luggage.

The legal speed of the packet boats was slow, traveling about 80 miles in twenty-four hours. Travel prices varied. In 1835, the rate for passengers was five cents for a mule-pulled boat—that included meals and lodging. An example of the length of time it took to travel by packet: the trip of 363 miles from Albany to Buffalo took nine days. Then Eunice would need to take a carriage to the packet boat landing.

For Eunice to travel back and forth from Troy, New York, on a packet boat and carriage was difficult as well as impractical to visit her family. Instead, she spent the holidays with Catherine Cody and her family. Catherine was a fellow student whose father was a prominent attorney in the Troy area. Elisha Cody was an up-and-coming professional, and romance began to bloom.

The courtship took three to four years. Eunice and Elisha were married in 1841 and moved to Seneca Falls, the hub of women's suffrage. Elisha was a brilliant man who shared Eunice's passion for science and advocacy of women's rights. It was a case of like minds think alike.

Both husband and wife held patents. Two that belonged to Eunice were improving paper-making machines and inventing a filling for shoes between the insoles and outer soles for keeping dry. Elisha was a judge whose specialty was patent law. When he was appointed commissioner of patents by President Lincoln in 1869, Elisha, Eunice and their two daughters relocated to Washington, D.C., and began a different lifestyle, one of politics.

They were active participants in the original 1848 Women's Rights Convention. Both of them signed the historic and famous Declaration of Sentiments. Of the one hundred signatures, Eunice's name was fifth. Surprisingly, thirty-two of the signatories were men, and Elisha was quite proud to add his name to the list of gentlemen who were in favor of the movement. Male support was crucial to the cause.

Though Eunice's name is not a household one, many of her achievements were the forerunners of today's science discoveries, such as the "greenhouse effect." She stood in the shadows of history-making women such as Abigail Adams, Lucretia Mott, Cady Stanton and Elizabeth Blackwell.

Elisha died in 1883, and Eunice followed five years later. She was a trailblazer for other female scientists making one footprint at a time. Recognition for her work finally came when she was nominated for induction into the Seneca Falls Women's Hall of Fame in Seneca Falls, New York, in 2021.

BLANCHE STUART SCOTT
(1884–1970), "TOMBOY OF THE AIR"

Hammondsport

S top this child from driving a dangerous vehicle!" So ordered the
Rochester, New York City Council in 1902.

That child was Blanche Stuart Scott, who was a daredevil even at age
thirteen. She was fascinated with activities that involved moving fast, and
she could be seen speeding around the streets of Rochester at thirty miles an
hour, scaring both horses and pedestrians.

Blanche was the apple of her dad's eye, but when he died, her mother
took over the family business in hopes of transforming Blanche into a lady.
It didn't work.

Instead, she headed to New York City, where she became an automobile
salesperson—very likely the first woman to do so. Blanche took every
opportunity to make a name for herself. She sent a letter to the Willys-
Overland Motor Company suggesting it sponsor her in a transcontinental
driving trip to promote and prove that women could drive cars.

On May 16, 1910, Blanche set off from New York City, beginning a
historic trip from the Atlantic Ocean to the Pacific. Thousands of people
lined Fifth Avenue to see the Lady Overland in a moment of history. The
fancy car had twenty-five horsepower, acetylene lamps for night driving,
spare tires and a cylinder of compressed air in case of a flat. What it didn't
have was a trunk. Early cars were not designed with them until years later,
making the Lady Overland a novelty that attracted a lot of attention.

Blanche had a female companion, a journalist, who recorded their
progress daily, with the big newspapers running pages of photographs and

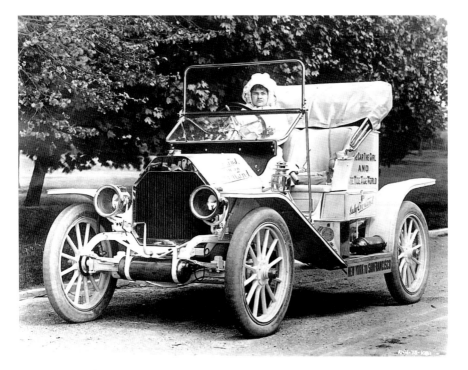

Blanche in her Overland automobile during her cross-country trek. Author's collection.

stories every Sunday. The cross-country route was not a straight line but a zigzag course because Blanche had to drive to and from each of the 175 Overland agencies. The extra stops doubled the mileage from 3,000 to 6,000 miles—quite a feat, since there were only 218 miles of paved roads at the time.

The trip involved many challenges: everything from rutted, unpaved roads, a threatening wild cat and rivers without bridges. But there was one obstacle no one had planned or foreseen: a call from Mother Nature. An escort car, with all men, preceded the Lady Overland in case of trouble. There was just one problem. The two women couldn't risk the embarrassment of stopping by the wayside to use it as a bathroom. Being resourceful, Blanche came up with a solution on an overnight stop. After passing by a drugstore window display, she bought a stomach pump with a wide funnel attached to a long hose. By cutting a hole in the floorboard of the car and inserting the pump and funnel, she created a portable potty. The reporters were mystified to say the least. How could two women drive all day without stopping? Blanche answered them by saying, "Cast-iron kidneys, boys."

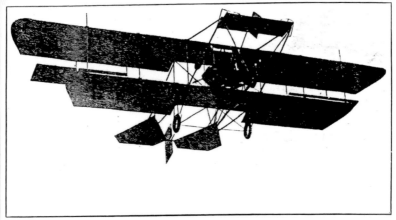
Advertisement for an exhibition promoting the Glenn L. Martin Company featuring
Blanche Scott. *Author's collection.*

Blanche loved the limelight, and when the opportunity came to ride in a two-seater plane for a news stunt, she jumped at the chance to fly in an airplane. It was a relief when the event didn't happen due to severe stormy weather.

When a press agent for the Glenn Curtiss Flying Exhibition Company suggested that Blanche could promote Curtiss aircraft in the same way that she had done for Overland cars, Blanche seized the opportunity, saying, "Wonderful idea!" Never mind that she didn't know how to fly.

Aviation was literally just getting off the ground. There was intense rivalry between the Wright brothers and Glenn Curtiss to obtain patents for plane designs. Flying machines were a huge novelty and drew large crowds. Adding Blanche to the Curtiss team would be real one-upmanship. There was just one hitch: Curtiss was livid with rage. He believed that a woman's place was in the home and not in the air. He told her that if she were killed or injured, it would set aviation back twenty years. Her smiling reply was, "I have a contract."

Reluctantly, Curtiss began training Blanche to fly in a single-seat biplane. It looked like a huge tricycle with transparent wings and a propeller in the rear. The pilot sat between the wings and behind the pilot's seat. If the plane crashed, the motor could break loose and decapitate the pilot. The position was aptly called the "undertaker's chair." Blanche's lessons consisted of taxiing up and down the field with Curtiss shouting instructions until the day when she removed the block of wood holding the plane down on the ground, and up and away Blanche flew, much to the annoyance of Curtiss.

For her first flying lesson, Blanche had a special tailored suit made. It was designed to keep the suit's ankle-length pleated skirt with four yards of material at the hemline from flying over her head. A bicycle clip did the trick.

Blanche became the poster girl for women flyers. Handbills declared her the "Tomboy of the Air" because she performed daring aerial stunts that thrilled exhibition audiences. When she soloed in 1910, licenses for pilots didn't exist. A year later, the Aero Club of America began to issue them. To her regret, Blanche followed Curtiss's advice; he didn't think they were necessary. That case of poor judgment cost Blanche the claim of being the first licensed American woman pilot. That credit went to Harriet Quimby.

The summer of 1911 was filled with Blanche performing exhibition flying at state fairs, racetracks, carnivals and anywhere there was a crowd and a place to land. Meanwhile, Blanche had solved the problem of what to wear while flying. The numerous petticoats under full-length dresses were too hazardous, even with bicycle clips. She had a New York City designer

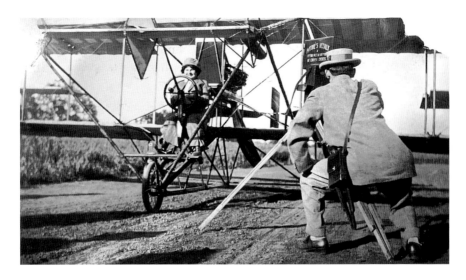

Above: Blanche filming a
"Pathé's Weekly."
Author's collection.

Right: Blanche posing in
lucky red sweater at the
Emeryville Race Track,
Oakland, California, 1912.
Author's collection.

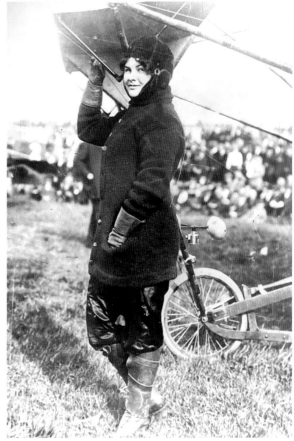

fashion a brown satin suit with baggy knee breeches. Her accessories were high boots, a brown plush helmet, earmuffs and gauntlets. It was daring attire for the times, but her full-cut bloomers were manageable for flying.

Blanche was superstitious and completed her jaunty outfit with an old red sweater, which she always wore. She believed it was a symbol of a guardian angel who protected her from harm. That guardian would be put to the test several times.

Harriet Quimby, one of the early female pilots on the exhibition circuit, crossed paths with Blanche several times, but the last time turned into a tragedy.

Fifteen aviators were participating in an aerial show at Squantum Airfield in Massachusetts, on July 1, 1912. Harriet and Blanche were the only women competing. Harriet was flying a seventy-horsepower French Bleriot two-seater that was quite unstable. Balance was maintained by strategically placing a bag of sand to keep the center of gravity. William Willard, a large man, sat in the passenger seat behind Harriet. He had been warned to sit perfectly still but leaned forward anyway to speak to Harriet. His movement upset the balance of the plane, which nose-dived into a marsh. Both were killed instantly.

Blanche was in the air when it happened and knew something terrible had happened to Harriet, but she was unable to land because of the crowd on the runway. She had to circle the field five times. The accident unnerved her but didn't discourage her from flying. Unfortunately, the incident just gave fuel to the naysayers who didn't believe women should fly. But Blanche was not out of gas just yet, nor was she spared from risks.

During her career, three attempts were made on her life. The first two times a mechanic deliberately dropped a wrench into the propellers, causing them to shatter in air. The man resented the fact that Blanche was permitted to fly and he hadn't been. The third time, a woman pulled a gun on her. She claimed that she was the widow of a pilot who had been killed and Blanche was the reason because the man wanted to marry her. In all three times, she believed her lucky red sweater came to her rescue.

Promotional handbills named her "Tomboy of the Air" for the daring stunts she performed, especially her "death dive," when she flew under bridges.

Memorial Day 1913 was a fateful day. Blanche was flying in an air exhibition in Madison, Wisconsin. It was a warm day, and she didn't wear her lucky red sweater. She took off as usual, but at two hundred feet the throttle wire snapped. In circumstances similar to Quimby's, her plane took a nosedive into a swamp, throwing Blanche from the plane and breaking

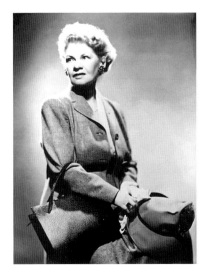

Formal portrait of Blanche in her later years, 1955. *Author's collection.*

forty-one bones in her body. She spent eight months in a cast. She believed that the mishap was sabotage because the cut on the wire was a clean one; her missing sweater could also have been responsible for the terrible mishap.

Despite her severe injuries, Blanche wasn't ready to give up her passion for flying, but her long recovery took a toll on her, and she retired from active flying in 1916.

Throughout her flying days, Blanche achieved many historic aviation "firsts." Among them were: first and only woman taught by Glenn Curtiss; first woman stunt flyer; first long-distance flight by a woman; first woman test pilot. On September 6, 1948, she became the first American woman to fly in a jet plane, piloted by Chuck Yaeger, the man who broke the sound barrier. Blanche was a passenger and loved every minute of the flight.

Blanche entered a new phase of her life. She acquired materials for the U.S. Air Force Museum and went to Hollywood and worked as a script writer for film studios for fourteen years.

She was quoted in the *New York Herald* on July 16, 1911: "Women should wake up and take a serious, intelligent, articulate, practical interest in what makes the world tick." And she did.

MARY CLARK THOMPSON
(1835–1923), "SHARE THE WEALTH"

Naples

In the 1800s, few women could call themselves entrepreneurs, but Mary Clark Thompson was an exception.

People might think she was born with a silver spoon in her mouth, but that wasn't the case. Her father was a farmer who became interested in politics and was elected Ontario County sheriff in 1837. The family moved to Canandaigua and also ran a hardware store.

Mary was the third child of five and was educated in village schools and attended the Ontario Female Seminary, a leading institution of the time.

Wealth didn't come her way until she married Frederick Ferris Thompson on June 17, 1857. They met at an event in Albany, the New York State capital, hosted by Mary's father, Myron, who had been elected the governor of New York State. Frederick was the son of John Thompson, a famous and well-to-do New York banker. Frederick followed in his father's footsteps and was a founder of the First National Bank of New York. Politics would play a role throughout their lives.

The couple's primary residence was on Madison Avenue in New York City, but they spent their summers at Mary's childhood home in Canandaigua. In 1863, the Thompsons purchased a three-hundred-acre farmstead from the Hoeberten family, who called the property Sonnenberg ("sunny hill" in German) for a small town in Germany, and the Thompsons kept the name.

In 1885, they tore down the existing farmhouse and replaced it with a forty-room Queen Anne–style mansion. Sonnenberg was on its way toward becoming a national treasure with nine formal gardens, aviaries and a thirteen-thousand-square-foot glass greenhouse complex.

Two of Mary's favorites were the Rose Garden and the Blue and White Garden. The Rose Garden featured thousands of new varieties in shades of crimson, pink and white, but not everything was coming up roses. The Blue and White Garden had lilies, forget-me-nots and larkspur. Sonnenberg was a prime example of a grand mansion with its many gardens. However, she didn't limit her interests to flowers: she also had a mushroom cellar constructed, and there were other gardens devoted to vegetables, melons, grapes and a children's garden for the community to share.

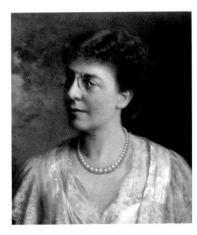

Mary Clark Thompson. *Courtesy of UR Medicine Thompson Health.*

Having no children of their own, and being financially comfortable, the Thompsons had the time and means to share their wealth to benefit others. They did so with monetary gifts to a lengthy list of organizations and institutions, large and small: they were the epitome of philanthropists. Mary was a founder of the Metropolitan Museum of Art and a contributor to the Bronx Zoo.

Supporting education was important to the couple, and they made substantial donations to major institutions. Some of those that benefited from their generosity included Williams College, Vassar College and Teacher's College (now Columbia University).

Mary didn't neglect local organizations but gave generously to the community where she lived. Notable beneficiaries were Canandaigua's Woodlawn Cemetery Chapel, Wood Library (Canandaigua), the city post office, a retirement home named for her parents, Clark Manor and the Ontario County Historical Society.

Probably the couple's most significant contribution was the establishment of F.F. Thompson Hospital in 1903. Named for her husband, it became the core of medical services for the Canandaigua area, then and now.

When Frederick died in 1889 at age sixty-two, Mary continued to make Canandaigua her summer home while traveling the world collecting ideas for the numerous flowerbeds and fine objects d'art. Each year, 1,500 annuals were planted.

In 2006, Sonnenberg Gardens and the Mansion were purchased by the New York State Office of Parks, Recreation and Historic Preservation, making it one of the few state-owned estates in the country. The arrangement helped stabilize the operations of the park, enabling it to open to thousands of visitors every year.

Mary's accolades were widespread and often unusual. For example, in 1920, she was awarded the Cornplanter Medal, named for multiple contributions to the State (New York) Museum in Albany and her support of preservation of the history of Native Americans, especially the Iroquois.

In 1921, she was awarded the eponymous Mary Clark Thompson Medal by the American Academy of Sciences for her commendable support of geology and paleontology. The award was originally presented every three years with a prize of $15,000. From 2017 on, it has been awarded alternatively with the Daniel Giraud Elliot Medal in Evolution of Earth and Life with a $20,000 prize, also for geology and paleontology.

In 1972, Sonnenberg Gardens Inc. was chartered by an act of Congress to preserve the mansion and gardens for display to the public. Mary would have, no doubt, been pleased. Though she was fairly healthy for her age at eighty-seven, her death was sudden, well one day and dead the next on July 28, 1923. The day of her funeral service, local businesses closed for the day out of respect. Her philanthropic endeavors left a legacy that benefited untold causes. She was the embodiment of "sharing one's wealth."

ERMA HEWITT
(1882–1970), "JEWELRY ARTISAN"

Bloomfield

W omen have had a love affair with jewelry from ancient times to the present. From Cleopatra to bling-sporting Hollywood stars, the larger, rarer, more expensive the gems, the better.

In the early 1800s, Manhattan was the hub of the jewelry district, with one name setting the benchmark for diamonds and luxury jewelry: Tiffany & Co.

Founded in 1837 by Charles Lewis Tiffany, the famous robin egg–blue box would turn many a head and warm the recipient's heart. The cachet of the name continues today.

In contrast to the glitz, there was a young woman whose jewelry creations were equally stunning. Her name is unknown to most people, but her contributions to the art of making jewelry with metals were distinctive and exceptional. That woman was Erma Hewitt. From farm girl to jewelry artisan, her techniques for incorporating metals with gems into broaches, rings and bracelets with her exquisite sense of design made her work unique. She even fashioned tiny links for necklace chains wound with silk cords that were popular at the time. She also turned her hands to carving ivory for adornments.

After graduating from high school, Erma taught school for a few years in Honeoye Falls, New York, before attending Pratt Institute in Brooklyn. That was just the beginning of a stellar career. Teaching would be a focus throughout her lifetime, as it was with her other three sisters, but her specialty subject was far from typical: it was making jewelry with metals.

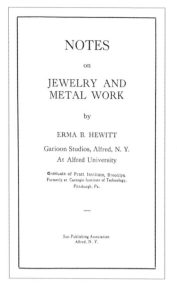

NOTES

on

JEWELRY AND
METAL WORK

by

ERMA B. HEWITT

Garioon Studios, Alfred, N. Y.

At Alfred University

Graduate of Pratt Institute, Brooklyn
Formerly at Carnegie Institute of Technology,
Pittsburgh. Pa.

—

Sun Publishing Association
Alfred, N. Y.

Erma Hewitt's important volume on the craft of jewelry and metal work. *Author's collection.*

She attributed her fascination with jewelry to chance. One day when she was walking past one of the Pratt classrooms, loud pounding drew her attention. When she realized that the noise came from students making bowls and jewelry, she was hooked.

Her coursework was silversmithing, jewelry and chasing. (Metal jewelry chasing is used to create dimensional works of art, mostly silver. The metal is raised by hammering from the back of the object to fabricate an image on the front.) Following her time at Pratt, she received training at the Rhode Island School of Design and worked in a studio in New York City for three years.

The next progression in her career was a position at the Carnegie Institute of Technology in Pittsburgh, Pennsylvania, where she taught metal and jewelry in the Art Department for nine years. But it was in 1924 that her talent and artistry peaked and was recognized. She accepted a job offer at Alfred University as an instructor in metalworking. Two events occurred during that time that brought attention to her work and shone a light on her creativity.

While she wrote some modest articles about her artwork, it was a small book (forty-two pages) published by Alfred that became the gold standard for directions in working with metals and jewelry. *Jewelry and Metal Work* became *the* textbook, with detailed step-by-step methods that are so precise that it can still instruct craftspeople today.

Her second achievement was an exhibit of her work in the Craft Building of the 1933 World's Fair in Chicago, which brought major attention to her handiwork.

Surprisingly, the accomplished woman whose creations were coveted by many didn't wear her own jewelry. In an interview in the 1967 *Daily Messenger*, Erma modestly said: "I've had a wonderful time working with jewelry. It may seem strange but although I loved to work with it, it never occurred to me to wear jewelry." (Not even her own!)

During her thirty years of teaching at Pratt, she also maintained a gift shop for twenty years. People were known to line up outside the shop into the

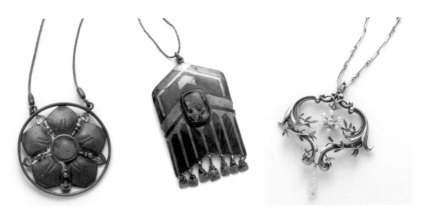

Hewitt Jewelry. *Courtesy of the Ontario County Historical Society.*

evening hours just to purchase one of her prized pieces. Her students were lucky and so were her fans who were fortunate enough to obtain one of her prized pieces.

Nine of her pieces are in the collections of the Ontario County Historical Society.

Erma retired at the age of eighty-four when poor health forced her to return to live with her maiden sisters in Bloomfield. The saying, "You can take the girl out of the farm, but you can't take the farm out of the girl," applies to Erma. She kept close touch with her family, often visiting her parents and siblings.

The diary that her sister Carrie kept provides an inside peek into their daily activities and farm chores. On July 7, 1965, she wrote: "The central operator called and tried to teach us how to use the dial [telephone] system. Will have to get used to it."

Another entry, on February 4, 1966, recounted: "Just before dark Mr. Dolan asked us if we knew we had a bird in the front room. We went in, there was a pheasant that had flown right through the upper sash of the north east window. He replaced the glass the next day, grabbed the bird and threw it out the (new) window."

Erma was a strong professional woman in a time when women were expected to remain at home and look after the household.

Her precision with line, form and color made her a true artist. Sadly, she died in 1970 when she was struck and killed by a car as she crossed the road near her house.

LOUISE SCHERBYN
(1898–2003), "OFF TO THE RACES"

Waterloo

Start your engines! With the wave of a flag, an automobile race is off to a flying start. In today's world, racing is a wildly popular sport. Companies often sponsor teams, and fans will pick a favorite driver. In the 1930s, racing was much different. Women drivers were an oddity. Any ladies who dared to race engine-powered vehicles were considered scandalous—and, in fact, shocking—especially women riding on motorcycles. That didn't faze Louise Scherbyn one bit.

Many a couple has endured harsh words while trying to involve each other in the activities one or the other liked. In the case of Louise, her husband, George, tried to teach her to shoot and fish, but neither sport "took." George didn't give up, and it was while they were on their honeymoon that he suggested she try riding a motorcycle. There were instant sparks: Louise had found her second love, motorcycles! And when a friend took her for a ride in a sidecar, she was hooked.

George cautioned her never to speed, and if she did, he would toss her into jail and leave her there. One incident came very close to making that happen.

To say that Louise was an attraction is an understatement. Riding an all-white Indian Scout motorcycle outfitted with white saddlebags and a foxtail flying in the breeze was her trademark. A matching custom-made white suit with white knickers, knee-high white boots and helmet completed the outfit, making her hard to miss.

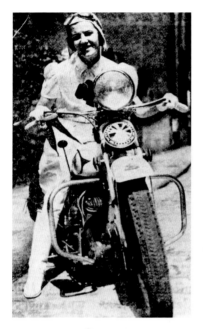

Louise on one of her motorcycles in 1939. *From the* Democrat & Chronicle, *August 19, 1939.*

Every Sunday, Louise rode from Rochester, New York, to Waterloo, New York, to visit her parents. At that time, in the 1930s, she believed she was the only female motorcyclist on the road. She loved being noticed, and the ride went along smoothly until Louise saw a state trooper in her mirror following her. She knew she wasn't speeding; the limit was forty-five miles per hour, but the trooper pulled her over. All Louise could think about was George's admonition about jail. When Louise timidly looked up and saw that the trooper was grinning, she suspected she wasn't in trouble. He confessed that the other troopers had told him to watch for this daredevil woman on a white motorcycle so he could get a look at her. No doubt she was both flattered and relieved that she wasn't going to jail.

Louise's enthusiasm spread from endurance racing to stunt riding to organizing women's motorcycle clubs. In 1940, the Motor Maids of America was established as the first all-female riding club. They traveled as a group to perform at events and held conventions. She arranged for an All-Girl Motorcycle Show in Waterloo, which led from one parade to another.

Word spread about this crazy woman who not only rode a bike but also performed stunts attired in ladylike fashion wearing white gloves. One feat in particular was a crowd favorite: Louise would lie down backward across the front fender of the bike while another woman drove. Risky at best.

In 1952, she said, "There should be a worldwide organization for all women motorcyclists." Louise stepped up to the plate and started one. The Women's International Motorcycle Association is the oldest existing motorcycle club for women, with chapters in thirty-nine countries.

She was member number six in WIMA and served as its secretary, designing decals and uniform decorations. In her secretarial position, she received postcards from women across America. Many of them had their number of motorcycle miles scrawled across the back.

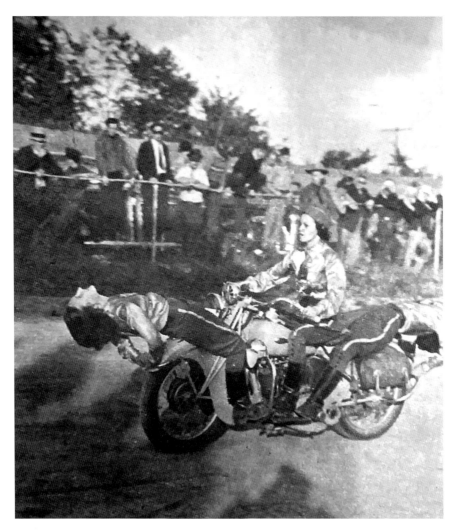

Louise in a daredevil stunt. *Author's collection.*

Louise and her fellow cyclists often encountered unexpected situations, like the time she and another female biker started on a five-hundred-mile jaunt to Canada. It was a hot day, and the women were dressed in light clothing, but before long the temperature dropped and rain set in. Soaked, cold and hungry, they kept going until they reached the only restaurant for miles, desperately in need of hot coffee. It was just their luck that the owner couldn't serve them any because a skunk had fallen into the well.

Louise was far from camera shy, and despite her demure looks, she was not above playing pranks. She planned a "hare-and-hound race" for the Newark, New Jersey Club. The fifty-mile course was scattered with obstacles, but as the organizer of the chase and therefore, "the hare," Louise had a two-minute head start and sped off. When she reached the fifty-mile marker, she pulled a fast one. As she had planned, she roared her Indian Scout up a plank into the back of a truck, pulled a tarp over her bike and herself and lay there for hours trying not to laugh out loud as the hounds roared by searching for her.

At other times, her feisty nature surfaced. During one interview, someone dared to ask her age, and Louise sternly scolded the person: "Don't you go saying how old I am. Folks will say an old lady has no business fooling with motorcycles but I feel like a young chicken."

Evidently, she didn't mind answering the sensitive question of how she kept her girlish figure. She shyly admitted that the scales never tipped more than 100 to 104 pounds and she never felt better in her life.

But sadly, arthritis would cripple her hands and hamper her ability to ride, but she wasn't done with motorcycles. One record claims that by 1951, Louise had ridden a total of 225,000 miles without ever having an accident. Perhaps that was due to her lucky rabbit's foot that she always carried for good luck. She also claimed that she was the first woman to ride a motorcycle to the far north of Canada to the undeveloped Temagami Lake territory. The dirt and gravel roads didn't slow Louise down.

Louise could have been the poster girl for motorcycles. She was loyal to Indian brand cycles. She owned three and kept her first one in her basement. Among her many accolades as a pioneering female motorcyclist, she was inducted into the Indian Motorcycle Museum Hall of Fame in 1988. When she retired, she donated a bike to the Indian Motorcycle Museum in Springfield, Massachusetts.

For a woman devoted to Indian motorcycles, it's amusing that she had a Harley Davidson tattoo in a prominent place. Her most noteworthy contribution was establishing the Women's International Association in 1950. It was the first organization to recognize all women in the sport. Branches sprang up around the world, and today it is the largest motorcycle association for women, thanks to Louise.

Louise and George's involvement with biking and bikers didn't end when her thirty years of stunt performing were over. They opened up their home in Waterloo to cyclists, providing a mecca for riders to share stories and remembrances and check out her collection of over three hundred toy cycles.

As an enthusiastic scrapbooker, Louise filled box after box with memorabilia, ticket stubs, newspaper clippings, correspondence and trophies. Those scrapbooks are housed in the Waterloo Historical Society Archives.

Louise's love affair with two-wheeled machines came to an end on June 18, 2003. The motto of the American Motorcycle Association is the perfect description for Louise: "To promote the motorcycle lifestyle and protect the future of motorcycling." Louise Scherbyn lived to be over one hundred years old, having devoted her life to that mission, and she left tire tracks for other women to follow.

Louise is buried in the St. Francis Cemetery in Phelps, near Waterloo.

NARCISSA PRENTISS WHITMAN (1808–1847), "MIXED BLESSINGS"

Prattsburg

Narcissa was a woman with a mission—literally. She was born in Prattsburgh, New York, where her father, Stephen, cleared land for a small farm and later took over the operation of a gristmill and a sawmill. As a carpenter, he used lumber from the mill to build a modest frame house for his growing family, and grow it did. Narcissa was the third of nine children and the oldest of five daughters.

The region where the family lived was known as the "burned-over district," not because of wildfires but due to another kind of fire, evangelistic fervor. In the nineteenth century, fiery sermons, public confessions of sin and collective conversions were rampant throughout the area.

The minister of the Prattsburgh Presbyterian Church was delighted to see weeping and trembling among the people attending his revival in 1819. At the end of the fire-and-brimstone experience, he welcomed fifty-nine new members. One of them was eleven-year-old Narcissa. At age sixteen, a second spiritual awakening convinced her that her true calling was to be a missionary.

For a woman of her generation, Narcissa was well educated. She was among the first class of women to attend the Franklin Academy, a church-affiliated secondary school in Prattsburgh. She completed a twenty-one-week course in 1828 and returned for a second term two years later.

Then, Marcus Whitman entered her life. At age twenty-one, he left his family business to apprentice himself to become a physician. He worked as a country doctor in Pennsylvania and Canada before joining the Wheller Presbyterian Church (nine miles south of Prattsburgh). He served as a trustee, an elder and a Sunday School superintendent.

What he really wanted was to receive a commission as a medical missionary, but the American Board of Commissioners for Foreign Missions (ABCFM) rejected his application in 1834 because of concerns about his health. Five months later, he met Reverend Samuel Parker, who was on a one-man crusade to send missionaries to Indians in the American West. Despite the ABCFM's concerns and lack of enthusiasm for Marcus's request to establish a mission in Oregon Country, they agreed to sponsor his efforts if he could raise the money himself. He did so by touring churches and asking for donations, arriving in Wheeler, Oregon, in 1834.

Whitman's enthusiasm was matched with Parker's readiness to have someone accompany him on an exploratory trip to the West to scout possible mission sites. Marcus's letter to the board on December 2, 1834, reassured them that his health had restored so much that it would not offer any impediment. Little did he know that other obstacles would threaten his life.

Parker left Wheeler and traveled to the newly settled village of Amity, forty-five miles west. The Prentiss family had moved there in 1834 so Narcissa's father could get work as a carpenter. Parker used the log schoolhouse and church as a platform to plead for missionaries to go to Oregon Country.

He believed that his prayers were answered when he learned that Narcissa Prentiss, a single woman, had volunteered to go to Oregon as a missionary so they could go as husband and wife. It didn't matter that they had never met. Marcus arrived in Amity on February 22, 1835, and they were engaged the next day. Since Marcus had agreed to accompany Parker, it would be a year before the couple would see each other again. In the meantime, the board offered them missionary positions as soon as they were married. Marcus's hope and Narcissa's dream were about to become real.

The deadline for leaving was looming, and Marcus was desperate to find another couple to go with them. He finally persuaded Henry Spaulding, a Presbyterian minister, and his wife, Eliza, to go to Oregon Country instead of the Osage mission in western Missouri. Wasting no time, Narcissa and Marcus were married on February 18, 1836, and the two couples left for Oregon immediately to begin their missionary duties. Narcissa and Eliza were the first white women to cross the Rocky Mountains. The three-thousand-mile journey would test their courage, stamina and faith.

At first, Narcissa enjoyed the beautiful landscapes. She wrote in her journal on March 26, 1836, that she was in good spirits and looked forward to the journey going well, but the 1,900 miles of mountains and deserts that lay ahead of them quickly changed into hazardous conditions. Their small missionary party made a practical decision to join the American Fur Company's caravan of seventy people for safety's sake.

When they stopped at the first Indian village, Narcissa and Eliza were the first white women the Indians had ever seen, and they were either baffled, skittish or fearful or all three. When the caravan stopped for a week at Fort William (later known as Wyoming), the women had a chance to wash their clothes for the first time in months. Narcissa met some Pawnee Indians and thought they were "noble." When some two hundred trappers, traders and Nez Perce gathered at the Green River, the two white women created quite a sensation. Narcissa entertained the leaders with a tea while Eliza focused on learning the Indian languages.

The Whitmans traveled ahead of the Spauldings and arrived at old Fort Walla Walla, a trading post on the Columbia River. Narcissa was in awe of the comforts there: soft chairs, fresh food, even salmon. They took the opportunity to visit Fort Vancouver, just three hundred miles down the Columbia River. The fort was the headquarters of the Hudson Bay Company, which was large enough to house forty buildings, including a school, a chapel and even a library. The fort had become a thriving commercial and supply station.

When both couples reached Fort Vancouver, they decided to establish separate missions. Spaulding chose a site in Nez Perce territory while the Whitmans settled in Cayuse territory called "People of the Place of the Rye Grass." The name sounded pleasant enough, but the Cayuse were far from it. In spite of warnings about them, Whitman went ahead and farmed and provided medical care. Narcissa even set up a school for the Native American children. However, things did not bode well.

The mission was settling in as Marcus held church services while Narcissa taught school to the Natives. But the happy days were short-lived. Narcissa soon became repulsed by what she perceived as the dirty and lazy ways of the Indians. Worst of all, they rejected any religious messages.

The one bright spot in Narcissa's life was her daughter, Alice, but tragedy struck. Alice was only two years old when she went down to the riverbank to fill her cup with water. She fell in and drowned. Narcissa's bright spot was extinguished that day. She was overcome with grief and guilt, sinking into a deep depression and retreating into illness. She rarely

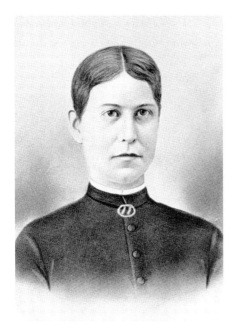

Portrait of Narcissa Prentiss Whitman, from
O.W. Nixon's *How Marcus Whitman Saved
Oregon. Courtesy of Wikimedia Commons.*

left her room and wondered if God was punishing her.

Without any children of their own, the Whitmans began to take in orphans whose parents had died on the Oregon Trail. Meanwhile, the ABCFM had decided to close the mission due to a lack of converts. Marcus immediately left for Boston, hoping to change their minds, but was unsuccessful. On his return in 1843, he helped lead the first "Great Migration," a wagon train of eight hundred or more pioneers heading West. Tensions between the Natives and the Whitmans reached a high level, forcing the Whitmans to forego any more missionary efforts and operate a hotel and trading post for white immigrants instead.

The strained relationship turned to brutal violence on November 29, 1847. The Cayuse resented the white settlers who brought infectious diseases. Because they lacked immunity, many Indians died from an epidemic of measles. They blamed the Whitmans, and on a fateful day when Marcus and Narcissa refused their demands for milk and medicine, a fatal attack took place. Marcus was struck on the back of the head with a tomahawk. Narcissa was whipped, shot and dumped in the mud outside their house. Twelve more white settlers were killed along with the ten orphans the Whitmans had taken in.

Narcissa and Marcus did not die in vain. Their legacy is commemorated with many historic markers: the Whitman Mission National Historic Site, a sculpture at the entrance to Whitman College and many schools that are named for them, including his hometown school Marcus Whitman Central School in Rushville, New York. It was Marcus's political influence that was significant in establishing the states of Oregon and Washington.

While Marcus is credited with leading hundreds of settlers along the Oregon Trail, he couldn't have accomplished all he did without Narcissa. Many of the details of their challenges and tribulations were provided by her journals and letters home. She received her own tribute in 1979 when the Narcissa Prentiss House was opened to the public in Prattsburgh. Both pioneers were inducted into the Steuben County Hall of Fame, Narcissa in 1976 and Marcus in 1977. In 1998, Narcissus was recognized by the New York Governor's Commission honoring the achievements of women.

They are buried side by side near the massacre site in Walla Walla.

CRYSTAL EASTMAN (1881–1928), "ADVOCATE"

Canandaigua

When most people hear the name Eastman they think of George Eastman, the man behind Eastman cameras, film and Kodak. He was an entrepreneur who donated millions to organizations. If Crystal Eastman had received the same attention and commercial success, her name might be known worldwide as well. However, this is not the case, nor is there a direct family connection.

When Crystal was two, her parents, Samuel Eastman and Annis Bertha Ford, moved the family from Massachusetts to Canandaigua. She was greatly influenced by their pursuits of women's suffrage and religion, but it was her mother who encouraged her passion for religion, and it would become a dominant part of the family's lives.

Her mother was one of the first women ordained as a Protestant minister in America, and she became a minister of the Congregational Church, as did her father. The two of them served as pastors at the Church of Thomas Beecher near Elmira, where Samuel and Annis became friends with the notable author Mark Twain. It was through the church that the Eastmans became friends with the famous author, and Crystal joined the group soon after.

At that time in New York State, there was an area labeled the "burned-over district"—not because of devastating fires but due to the heat over controversial women's issues that focused on abolitionism, religious beliefs, evangelism and even the Underground Railroad. It cut a wide swath between the Finger Lakes and Lake Erie. Preachers promised divine wrath and their sermons of "hell, fire and brimstone" left many women in tears or fainting.

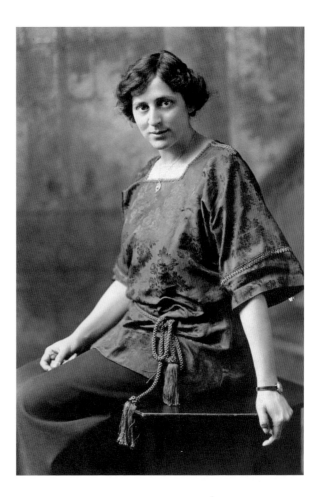

Eastman in 1914. *Courtesy of the Library of Congress.*

Her parents met at Oberlin College in Ohio and were married in 1875. Crystal's father suffered from a chronic illness due to severe pneumonia that he likely contracted during his stint in the Civil War. His health continued to wax and wane, which meant limited income for the family.

Her mother, Annis, began teaching in local schools by day and preaching at night. Due to her compelling sermonizing, she received offers to preach at area churches, increasing her popularity and bringing in some money.

Crystal pursued her interest in law and sociology and graduated from Vassar College in 1903. The next year, she received a Master of Arts degree in sociology from Columbia University. From there, she attended New York University Law School and graduated in 1907, the second in her class, a rare accomplishment for a woman in those days, but all that education was priming her for her future activism.

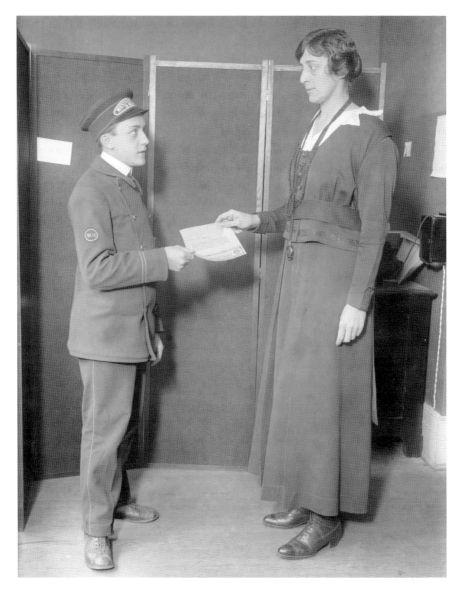

Crystal Eastman in 1915. *Courtesy of the Library of Congress.*

Her first job was investigating labor conditions for the *Pittsburgh Survey,* sponsored by the Russell Sage Foundation. Her report *Work Accidents and the Law,* published in 1910, became a classic that led to the first workers' compensation law, which she drafted when she was serving on a New York State commission.

Crystal's life wasn't all work; she was briefly married to Wallace Benedict, a longtime friend, and moved with him to Milwaukee, his hometown. But when her suffrage referendum there failed to pass, she returned to New York, ending their marriage in divorce in 1915 (supposedly because of his infidelities). But she didn't give up on romance and married her second husband, Walter Fuller, an English pacifist and editor. He had come to the United States to promote his four sisters' act of singing folksongs and to escape World War I.

She also organized the National Civil Liberties Union to protect conscientious objectors. During the war, Crystal joined Jane Addams and Lillian Wald and others in founding the Women's Peace Party and served as president of the New York chapter. Her peace efforts were her focus, and she became executor of the American Union Against Militarism, a lobby against profiteering from arms sales and military intervention.

Walter and Crystal had two children and shocked the country when she kept her own name and refused alimony because it would force mothers to depend on men financially. Plus, their living arrangements also caused consternation, as they kept separate households. She wrote a letter in response to her cynics titled *Marriage Under Two Roofs*, which claimed it created better sex.

Then, there was a third man in Crystal's life, her brother Max. The two siblings were close to each other, just two years apart. They lived together for a few years in New York City in Greenwich Village (at 27 West 11th Street) where there was a group of extreme activists that included Ernest Hemingway and Helen Keller; Crystal and Max fit right in. They put their beliefs together and co-founded and co-edited a radical journal on politics, art and literature called *The Liberator: The Journal of Revolutionary Progress* in 1918. It was a monthly socialist magazine that stirred up controversy; for example, they chose to publish it on Abraham Lincoln's birthday in 1918.

Even after the ratification of the Nineteenth Amendment, which gave women the right to vote, Crystal didn't slow down her campaign for gender equality.

Her speech "Now We Can Begin" became the testimonial for women's rights. During World War I, she was the leader of the women who founded the Woman's Peace Party of New York, which later was renamed Women's International League of Peace and Freedom (WILPF), the oldest peace organization still standing, with over one hundred branches in the United States. Crystal became the executive secretary.

There was one other significant association that Crystal helped organize: the American Civil Liberties Union (ACLU), which has become the watchdog for protecting Americans' rights under the Bill of Rights and is still active today. Unfortunately, Crystal never received the credit she deserved for her role in establishing the ACLU, due to differences within the party and her outspoken nature.

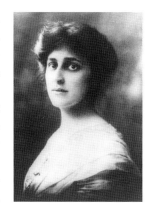

Portrait of Eastman. *Courtesy of the Library of Congress.*

During Woodrow Wilson's presidency, she served as attorney for the Commission on Industrial Relations, investigating occupational safety and health and earning her the title of "most dangerous woman in America." On the other hand, the editor of *The Nation* described her as "the voice of the working class."

From 1919 to 1921, when fears of communism, the "Red Scare," were rampant across the country, Crystal was blacklisted due to her radical activities as a pacifist, a feminist and an idealist. Put those attributes together, and you have one strong-willed woman who pursued equality and justice for women and the underdog.

Validation finally came her way when she was named to the National Women's Hall of Fame in Seneca Falls, New York, in 2000, in recognition of her efforts. As of 2021, she joined 303 other inductees, which at that time included Amelia Earhart, Amelia Bloomer, Maya Angelou and Marian Anderson. Margaret Mead was the first woman to be so honored.

Neither Crystal nor Walter lived long enough to fully appreciate their achievements. The couple sailed back and forth between England and the United States, but their reunion was short-lived: Walter died in 1927 from high blood pressure caused by stroke and overwork just nine months before Crystal. She died from nephritis at age forty-seven. She left behind her working-class voice, having earned her rightful place in the pursuit of women's equality. Her death left her two children, Jeffrey, eleven, and daughter, Annis, seven, without parents. Good friends took them in and finished raising the children.

BIBLIOGRAPHY

American Association for the History of Nursing. "Anna Caroline Maxwell." http://www.aahn.org.

Balin, Carole B. "Harriet Tubman and Sarah Hopkins Bradford: Women of Moral Courage from Auburn's Past." Auburn Seminary, https://auburnseminary.org.

Basinger, Jeanine. *Silent Stars*. New York: Alfred A. Knopf, 1999.

Bassett, Mark. "Breaking Tiffany's Glass Ceiling: Clara Wolcott Driscoll (1861–1994)." Cleveland Institute of Art. https://www.cia.edu.

Beale, Irene A. *Genesee Valley Women, 1743–1985*. Geneseo, NY: Chestnut Hill Press, 1985.

Boissoneault, Lorraine. "Amelia Bloomer Didn't Mean to Start a Fashion Revolution, But Her Name Became Synonymous with Trousers." *Smithsonian Magazine*, May 24, 2018. https://www.smithsonianmag.com.

Bradford, Sarah H. *The Moses of Her People: Harriet Tubman*. Secaucus, NJ: Citadel Press, 1961.

———. *Scenes in the Life of Harriet Tubman*. Auburn, NY: W.J. Moses, 1869.

Bridgeford-Smith, Jan. "Before He Was a Star! Humphrey Bogart and His Finger Lakes Summer." *Life in the Finger Lakes*, June 18, 2018. https://www.lifeinthefingerlakes.com.

Chapin, Becky. "Looking Back." *Finger Lakes Times*, December 10, 2022.

Cornell Daily Sun. "When Movies Were Made in Ithaca." October 27, 2011.

Couldrey, Viviane. *The Art of Louis Comfort Tiffany*. Edison, NJ: Wellfleet Press, 1989.

Cummins, Julie. *Tomboy of the Air: Daredevil Pilot Blanche Stuart Scott*. New York: HarperCollins, 2001.

Dahlquist, Marina, ed. *Exporting Perilous Pauline: Pearl White and the Serial Film Craze*. Chicago: University of Illinois Press, 2013.

———. "Pearl White." Women Film Pioneers Project. http://wfpp. columbia.edu.

Daily News. "Recollections of the Castile Water Cure." November 26, 2016. http://www.thedailynewsonline.com.

Doherty, Amy S., and David Tatam, eds. *Photography of Grace Woodworth: Outside the Common Lines*. Syracuse, NY: Syracuse University Press, 1986.

Drury, Clifford M. *Marcus and Narcissa Whitman and the Opening of the Old Oregon*. Seattle, WA: Northwest Interpretive Association, 1994.

Encyclopedia. "Greene, Dr. Cordelia A. (1831–1905)." encyclopedia.com.

Encyclopedia Britannica. "Elizabeth Blackwell: British American Physician." https://www.britannica.com.

Encyclopedia of Cleveland History. Case Western Reserve University. https://case.edu/ech/.

Engel, Helen, ed. *Remarkable Women in New York State History*. Charleston, SC: The History Press, 2013.

"A Fashion Revolution." *Victoriana Magazine*, September 29, 2014. www. victoriana.com/bloomer-costume.

Fox, Austin M. "Louise Blanchard Bethune: Buffalo Feminist and America's First Woman Architect." *Buffalo Spree*, Summer 1986. https://buffaloah. com.

Gable, Walt. "Looking Back—Part II: Seneca Falls Photographer Lived an Independent Life." *Finger Lakes Times*, August 3, 2020. https://www. fltimes.com.

Goddard, Charles W. *The Perils of Pauline*. Morris Plains, NJ: Murana Press, 2014.

Hays, Johanna. "Louise Blanchard Bethune: Architect Extraordinaire and First American Woman Architect Practiced in Buffalo, NY." Dissertation, Auburn University, 2007. http://www.auburn.edu.

"The Heroine of a Thousand Dangerous Stunts." *American Magazine*, September 1921.

HerrGesell, Leif. "Local History: More Than a Foote Note: The Story of Eunice Newton Foote." *Daily Messenger*, December 15, 2019.

History of American Women: Colonial Women | 18th–19th Century Women | Civil War Women. "Narcissa Whitman." https://www. womenhistoryblog.com.

Hofer, Margaret K. *The Lamps of Tiffany Studios: Nature Illuminated*. New York: New York Historical Society, 2016.

Home News (New Brunswick NJ). "Indian Motorcycle Museum Puts Visitors in Bygone Era." August 8, 1981.

Horta, Linda McCurdy. *Mary Clark Thompson and Her World*. Geneva, NY: Humphrey Press, 1984.

Huddleston, Amara. "Happy 200th Birthday to Eunice Foote, Hidden Climate Science Pioneer." NOAA, July 17, 2019. https://www.climate.gov.

Huett, Patrick. "Some Hollywood History Right Here in the Finger Lakes." Visit Finger Lakes, December 22, 2015. https://www.visitfingerlakes.com.

Hughes, James P. "Lights, Camera, Action…" *Life in the Finger Lakes Magazine*, May/June 2002.

Jacksonville University. "Top Nurses in History: Anna Caroline Maxwell." https://www.jacksonvilleu.com.

JCK, the Industry Authority. https://www.jckonline.com.

Jeffrey, Julie Roy. *Converting the West: a Biography of Narcissa Whitman*. Norman: University of Oklahoma Press, 1994.

Karwowski, Gerald. "Celebrating 175 Years: Western Printing." *Racine Post*. http://racinepost.blogspot.com.

Kastner, Jeffrey. "Clara Driscoll, One of the Guiding Lights Behind Tiffany's Success." *New York Times*, February 26, 2007. https://www.nytimes.com.

Klees, Emerson. *More Legends and Stories of the Finger Lakes Region*. Rochester, NY: Friends of the Finger Lakes Publishing, 1992.

———. *People of the Finger Lakes Region: The Heart of New York State*. Rochester, NY: Friends of the Finger Lakes Publishing, 1995.

Knox County Historical Society. *Amelia Bloomer: Exhibit*. Knhttp://www.knoxhistory.org.

Latrobe, Kathy, ed. "Etching." In *The Children's Literature Dictionary*, 65. New York: Neal-Schuman, 2002.

Levato, Ray. "The Mission of Narcissa Prentiss." *Life in the Finger Lakes*, July/August 2021.

Lickteig, Mary. *Amelia Bloomer*. Mankata, MN: Capstone Press, 1998.

Marcus, Leonard S. *How Golden Books Won Children's Hearts, Changed Publishing Forever, and Became an American Icon Along the Way*. New York: Golden Books, 2007.

Masoner, Liz. "A Brief History of Photography and the Camera." Spruce Crafts, July 6, 2023. www.thesprucecrafts.com.

McAlonie, Kelly Hayes. "Louise Blanchard Bethune." Pioneering Woman of American Architecture. https://pioneeringwomen.bwaf.org.

Menefee, David W. *The First Female Stars: Women of the Silent Era*. Westport, CO: Praeger, 2004.

Morry, Emily. "Ontario County Site Was Once a Health Mecca." *Democrat & Chronicle*, June 2, 2016.

National Park Service. "Amelia Bloomer." Women's Rights National Historical Park, https://www.nps.gov.

New York Historical Society. *A New Light on Tiffany: Clara Driscoll and the Tiffany Girls*. Exhibition, 2007.

Nimura, Janice P. *The Doctors Blackwell: How Two Pioneering Sisters Brought Medicine to Women and Women to Medicine*. New York: W.W. Norton, 2021.

Rochester Democrat & Chronicle. "Remarkable Women of the Finger Lakes." September 9, 1939.

———. "These Young Women Get Around." October 8, 1945.

Simmons, Christine Sommer. *The American Motorcycle Girls: A Photographic History of Early Women Motorcyclists*. West Nyack, NY: Parker House Publishing, 2009.

Slide, Anthony. "Pearl White." In *Silent Players: A Biographical and Autobiographical Study of 100 Silent Film Actors and Actresses*. Lexington: University Press of Kentucky, 2010.

Townsend, Wilma. "So Where's All the Old Stuff?" *OCHS Chronicles*, September 2011.

Vose, Courtney. "It Happened Here: Anna Maxwell." Health Matters. https://healthmatters.nyp.org.

Wemett, Laurel. "A Golden Era of Children's Books: Canandaigua Artist's Work Included in Little Golden Books Art Exhibit at MAG." *Daily Messenger*. https://www.mpnnow.com

———. "Mrs. Thompson's Conservatory." *Life in the Finger Lakes*. https://www.lifeinthefingerlakes.com.

Wharton Studio Museum. https://whartonstudiomuseum.org.

Wikipedia. "Amelia Bloomer." https://en.wikipedia.org/wiki/Amelia_Bloomer.

———. "Clara Driscoll (glass designer)." https://en.wikipedia.org/wiki/Clara_Driscoll_(glass_designer).

———. "Elizabeth Blackwell." https://en.wikipedia.org/wiki/Elizabeth_Blackwell.

———. "Eloise Wilkin." https://en.wikipedia.org/wiki/Eloise_Wilkin.

———. "Eunice Newton Foote." https://en.wikipedia.org/wiki/Eunice_Newton_Foote.

———. "Marcus Whitman." https://en.wikipedia.org/wiki/Marcus_Whitman.

———. "Mary Clark Thompson." https://en.wikipedia.org/wiki/Mary_Clark_Thompson.

———. "Mary Clark Thompson Medal." https://en.wikipedia.org/wiki/Mary_Clark_Thompson_Medal.

———. "Maud Humphrey." https://en.wikipedia.org/wiki/Maud_Humphrey.

———. "Pearl White." https://en.wikipedia.org/wiki/Pearl_White.

———. "Sarah Hopkins Bradford." http://en.wikipedia.org/wiki/Sarah_Hopkins_Bradford

———. "Whitman Mission National Historic Site." https://en.wikipedia.org/wiki/Whitman_Mission_National_Historic_Site.

Wilkin, Eloise, and Deborah Wilkin Springett. *The Golden Years of Eloise Wilkin*. New York: Random/Golden, 2004.

Women's International Motorcycle Association. "WIMA Pioneer Women: Louise Scherbyn." http://www.wimaworld.com.

Women's International Motorcycle Association Japan. "Our Founder: Louise Sherbyn (1903–2003)." http://www.wima.gr.jp/e_louise.html.

ABOUT THE AUTHOR

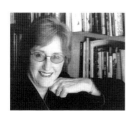 Julie Cummins is a nationally and internationally recognized authority on children's literature and library services. She was the coordinator of children's services for the New York Public Library for thirteen years and was the editor-in-chief of *School Library Journal.* Julie played an active leadership role in the American Library Association, including an elected term on the ALA Executive Board, chairing the Nominating Committee and serving twenty-two years on the ALA Council. In 2002, she received the Grolier Award, ALA's top award recognizing outstanding achievement in the profession for the stimulation and guidance of reading by children and young people, and in 2003, she received the Distinguished Service Award from the Association for Library Service to Children.

As an expert in children's literature and book illustration, she has chaired the Newbery and Caldecott Award committees as well as ALA's Notable Children's Book Committee and the Schneider Family Book Award. She has also served as a judge for the Boston Globe–Horn Book Award, the Jo Osborne Award for Humor in Children's Literature, the *New York Times* Best Illustrated Children's Books and the Society of Illustrators Children's Book Original Art exhibition.

In recent years, she has written her own children's books and books about children's literature:

The Inside-Outside Book of Libraries, illustrated by Roxie Munro (Dutton, 1996); Updated paperback edition (Random House, 2008)

Tomboy of the Air: Daredevil Pilot Blanche Stuart Scott (Harper, 2001)

Country Kid, City Kid, illustrated by Ted Rand (Holt, 2002)

Children's Book Illustration and Design, vols. 1 and 2 (PBC International, 1992 and 1996)

Women Daredevils: Thrills, Chills, and Frills, illustrated by Cheryl Harness (Dutton, 2008)

Sam Patch, Daredevil Jumper, illustrated by Michael Austin (Holiday House, 2009)

Women Explorers: Perils, Pistols, and Petticoats, illustrated by Cheryl Harness (Dial, 2012)

Flying Solo: How Ruth Elder Soared into America's Heart, illustrated by Malene Laugesen (Roaring Brook, 2013)

In addition, Julie has written numerous articles on children's books and children's services, presented speeches and workshops across the country, taught children's literature at four library schools and colleges and currently reviews children's books for two professional publications, *Booklist* and *Kirkus*.

Visit us at
www.historypress.com
....